Social responsibility in healthcare: Which application in Africa?

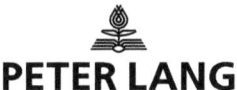

PETER LANG

Bruxelles - Berlin - Chennai - Lausanne - New York - Oxford

Intissar Haddiya

Social responsibility in healthcare: Which application in Africa?

The case of kidney disease management in African hospitals

Translated by Abdelhafid JABRI

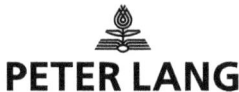

Bruxelles - Berlin - Chennai - Lausanne - New York - Oxford

Bibliographic information published by the Deutsche Nationalbibliothek.
The German National Library lists this publication in the German National
Bibliography; detailed bibliographic data is available on the Internet
at http://dnb.d-nb.de.

Library of Congress Cataloging-in-Publication Data
A CIP catalog record for this book has been applied for at the
Library of Congress.

Cover illustration: © iStock.com

© 2024 Peter Lang Group AG, Lausanne
Published by Peter Lang Éditions Scientifiques
Internationales - P.I.E., Brussels, Belgium

info@peterlang.com http://www.peterlang.com/

ISBN 978-2-87574-985-7
ePDF 978-2-87574-986-4
ePUB 978-2-87574-987-1
DOI 10.3726/b21372
D/2023/5678/65

All rights reserved.

All parts of this publication are protected by copyright.
Any utilization outside the strict limits of the copyright law, without the
permission of the publisher, is forbidden and liable to prosecution. This applies
in particular to reproductions, translations, microfilming, and storage and
processing in electronic retrieval systems.

Dedication

I would like to dedicate this book to my parents whom I thank heartily for their endless love and confidence in me. My father, Professor El Mostafa Haddiya , a symbol of rigor, integrity, and scientific probity, and my mother, Professor Naïma Agnaou , a bottomless source of wisdom and clear-sightedness have always believed in me and pushed me to be the best. I particularly would like to thank my husband, Professor Hicham Yacoubi, for his unshakable trust and for being my greatest inspiration, and my beloved children, Youssef and Rayan, for their patience. I deeply hope they are proud of me.

Acknowledgments

I am grateful to all the medical and paramedical staff at the participating hospitals across the continent for taking part in this study. My sincere thanks go to the nephrologists and professors of nephrology from all African regions for granting me unconditional access to their patients and teams, despite the long distances between us and the difficult pandemic situation, making their everyday experience at the hospitals harder. They believed in this work and kept repeating these encouraging words: "Go all the way with this study and make our voice heard! It's not that easy, but we're confident you can do it". These words were resonating deeply inside me during the various stages of this exciting scientific and human adventure. Their support allowed me to gain valuable insights into the healthcare systems of the African continent, identify weaknesses and deficiencies, and discuss solutions with my African friends and colleagues.

I would also like to extend my thanks to the epidemiologists and biostatisticians who accompanied me throughout this study. Their kindness, availability, and ability in managing a large amount of raw data deserve special recognition.

Finally, I would like to warmly thank all those who assisted, directly or indirectly, in the completion of this work, which I hope will meet the readers' expectations.

Preface

Social responsibility in healthcare is extremely important for the development of healthcare systems. It has gained much attention in the last few years, as it is often portrayed as one of the necessary responses to improve patient care in most developed countries. The healthcare sector should be guided by ethics to provide healthcare through socially responsible activities based on quality, equity, pertinence, and resource efficiency. In this context, governance is also of utmost importance, as managers of healthcare organisations are expected to shape their strategies and policies around social responsibility to improve health system performance. It is equally important to consider the social determinants of health to promote the health of the general population and establish socially responsible healthcare organisations.

Still, the concept of social responsibility has not significantly penetrated the non-profit healthcare environment. Besides, only a few studies have examined this concept in public hospitals, but no study has explored it from the perspective of internal stakeholders (doctors) and external stakeholders (patients) in the African continent. This survey aimed to address this research gap by investigating the factors affecting the social responsibility of African hospitals regarding in managing costly chronic diseases, using kidney disease as an example.

It is important to note that conducting such a survey requires accurate knowledge of the African continent from a socio-economic and healthcare perspectives. Most of the continent is characterised by poverty, mismanagement of healthcare funds, a lack of specialised infrastructure, and a shortage of qualified healthcare staff. All of these challenges hinder the provision of healthcare and pose significant challenges to the healthcare systems in Africa.

Intissar Haddiya

Table of contents

Abbreviations 15

Introduction 17

Part I: Social responsibility in healthcare

Chapter 1: Corporate social responsibility 23

Chapter 2: The values and obligations of healthcare organisations 37

Chapter 3: The ethical principles of social responsibility in healthcare 43

Chapter 4: The social responsibility of faculties of medicine 45

Chapter 5: The social determinants of health 47

Part II: The situation of health in Africa

Chapter 1: The context and situation of health in Africa 53

Chapter 2: African nephrology 81

Part III: Social responsibility in healthcare: An African-wide survey

Chapter 1: An African-wide survey 99

Chapter 2: Patients: The characteristics and perceptions of hospital social responsibility 101

Chapter 3: Nephrologists: The characteristics and perceptions of hospital social responsibility 143

Chapter 4: The factors influencing hospital social responsibility 169

Chapter 5: Ideas for enhancing hospital social responsibility in Africa 177

Conclusion 191

References 193

Table of contents 215

Abbreviations

AFRAN:	African Association of Nephrology
AKF:	Acute kidney failure
AMA:	American Medical Association
CHD:	Chronic hemodialysis
CI:	Confidence interval
CKD:	Chronic kidney disease
CKF:	Chronic kidney failure
CSP:	Corporate social performance
CSR:	Corporate social responsibility
ECA:	Economic Commission for Africa
ESKD:	End-stage kidney disease
FDA:	Food and Drug Administration
GDP:	Gross domestic product
GNP:	Gross national product
HD:	Hemodialysis
HIS:	Health information system
HIV:	Human immunodeficiency virus
ICU:	Intensive care unit
IMF:	International Monetary Fund
INN:	International non-proprietary name
ISN:	International Society of Nephrology
ISO:	International Organisation for Standardisation
KT:	Kidney transplantation
M/F:	(sex ratio) Male/Female
N/A:	Not available
NCDs:	Non-communicable diseases
NGO:	Nongovernmental organisation
NHANES:	National Health and Nutrition Examination Survey
PD:	Peritoneal dialysis
PMP:	Per million population
PPP:	Purchasing power parity
PRPP:	Production power parity
SD:	Standard deviation
UN:	United Nations
UNDP:	United Nations Development Programme

UNESCO:	United Nations Educational, Scientific and Cultural Organisation
UNICEF:	United Nations International Children's Emergency Fund
UNPF:	United Nations Population Fund
US:	United States
USAID:	United States Agency for International Development
USD:	US dollar
VS:	Versus
WHO:	World Health Organisation

Introduction

There are several definitions of corporate social responsibility (CSR). Simply put, it is the active involvement and participation of an organisation in actions that contribute to a more just society and safer environment. Thus, in current times of globalisation, adopting a social responsibility strategy could be a powerful tool for sustainability and for the survival of any business[1].

Unlike the traditional philanthropic view characterising businesses investing in charitable causes independent of their primary goals, successful corporate social responsibility (CSR) requires that various stakeholders come together to pursue common goals. Hence, CSR initiatives start with a solid strategic basis to relate corporate values to socially-based investments which, together, can enhance corporate performance and competitiveness[2].

Social responsibility has recently extended to other spheres of activity such as healthcare, especially health care provision, hospitals, and healthcare training centres. This new vision of social responsibility involves introducing a series of measures to improve access to healthcare for all, and enhance the quality and efficiency of healthcare services. This should be the case because human health remains a source of frequently asked and unresolved questions. Moreover, it is now acknowledged that the health status is determined not only by genetic and physiological factors, but also by various demographic, cultural, socio-economic, ecological, and health-related aspects that impact a population's health. This transcends the medical framework to become an evolving real project that considers the healthcare system parameters and the individuals' living conditions[3]. In fact, the social state acts in so far as the individual's socio-economic status, their working and living conditions, and the quality of their healthcare systems are the main determinants of their health and life expectancy. These social determinants influence the disease process along with

---

1 Pras B, Evrard Y, Roux E, *Market: études et recherches en marketing – Fondements, méthodes.* 3e éd. Dunod; 2003 p. 704.
2 Hammach M. *L'impact de la responsabilité sociale de l'entreprise sur l'implication organisationnelle des cadres salariés: cas du secteur de l'industrie agroalimentaire au Maroc.* Gestion et management. Conservatoire national des arts et métiers – CNAM, 2016. NNT: 2016CNAM1092.
3 La Rosa E et al. Social responsibility in health and the global health situation: towards new health and social indicators. *Revue de santé publique* 2007; 19(3): 217–227.

the biological and physiopathological factors. Moreover, the development of the social dimension of healthcare reflects the definition given to health by the World Health Organisation (WHO) in the Universal Declaration on Bioethics. According to the WHO, it is considered a foundation on which a new model of society can be built; a model which emphasises all the determinants of human well-being[4].

Thus, the social responsibility of healthcare systems is currently garnering increased attention around the world, as is the case with CSR. It is because the healthcare system has a direct impact on society and has, therefore, an ethical and moral obligation to be "socially responsible". In addition, many hospitals have shifted from providing essential health services to focussing on resource management, often due to financial constraints. Hence, the social responsibility of hospitals is attracting more attention, particularly in developing countries and transitional societies. Also, the social responsibility of healthcare organisations has been the focus of numerous studies worldwide. For instance, Brandao et al.[5], argued that hospitals should comply with the general ethical standards, promote anti-discrimination policies, and take part in national and international solidarity programmes to fulfil their social responsibility. For their part, Fottler et al.[6] stressed the importance of the social process within the overall healthcare process. Dharamsi et al.[7] concluded that social responsibility is a moral engagement which advances the medical profession and the underlying social contract. Furthermore, for Duggirala[8] and Rohini[9], social responsibility requires that every hospital functions as a facilitator of social well-being in accordance with the legal rules and regulations in force in order to meet society's expectations. It also requires that they take part in activities that promote human well-being

---

4   Rapport du Comité international de bioéthique de l'UNESCO (CIB) sur LA RESPONSABILITÉ SOCIALE ET LA SANTÉ, Publié par l'Organisation des Nations Unies pour l'éducation, la science et la culture. UNESCO 2010.
5   Brandão C et al. Social responsibility: a new paradigm of hospital governance?. *Health Care Analysis* 2013; 21(4): 390–402.
6   Fottler MD, Blair JD. *Challenges in health care management strategic perspectives for managing key stakeholders.* Jossey-Bass. 1990.
7   Dharamsi S, Ho A, Spadafora SM et al. The physician as health advocate: translating the quest for social responsibility into medical education and practice. *Academic Medicine* 2011; 86(9): 1108–1113.
8   Duggirala M. Patient-perceived dimensions of total quality service in healthcare. *Benchmarking An International Journal* 2008; 15(5): 560–583.
9   Rohini R. Social responsibility of hospitals: an Indian context. *Social Responsibility Journal* 2010; 6(2): 268–285.

and, more extensively, the quality of health care coupled with the legal, ethical, and philanthropic characteristics. These constitute the cornerstones of social responsibility of healthcare systems.

Although such studies provided a valuable insight into the nature of healthcare systems' social responsibility, only a few studies on this topic issuing from our continent or based on the perceptions of internal stakeholders (i.e., health professionals) or external stakeholders (i.e., patients) have been conducted. Thus, many believe that to improve the healthcare system, we need to understand how patients and caregivers see it[10].

It is therefore necessary to study social responsibility in healthcare in the African region from the perspective of patients and doctors so that scientific and technological progress will be fairly and equitably beneficial for patients, given the shocking disparities in healthcare access in many African countries. A concrete example of such disparities and inadequacies is the healthcare management of kidney disease in African regions. Besides poverty and illiteracy, several African countries are facing a shortage of healthcare facilities and human and material resources needed for the management of kidney disease, which remains common, serious, and costly[11]. Furthermore, the prevalence of nephropathy in this part of the world is closely linked to infections and a lack of awareness of preventive measures. Besides, without socially responsible healthcare systems that consider the social determinants of African populations as an integral part of patient management, neither the health situation in general nor the nephrological situation in particular will improve in our continent.

On the other hand, most works addressing CSR of healthcare providers mainly focussed on the philanthropic aspect and the socio-economic, charitable, or environmental actions, reducing the meaning of this concept to being a public health response or a support for the needy[12]. However, it should be noted that hospitals have firstly the professional obligation to fulfil their mission by providing accessible, equitable, affordable, and high-quality healthcare, and by taking appropriate initiatives to promote it. This aspect of professional responsibility of hospitals based on the promotion of a clinical approach and on the values of the patient, the caregiver, and the community is an essential

---

10 Liu W et al. How patients think about social responsibility of public hospitals in China?. *BMC Health Services Research* 2016; 16: 371.
11 Stanifer JW et al. The epidemiology of chronic kidney disease in sub-Saharan Africa: a systematic review and meta-analysis. *The Lancet. Global Health* 2014; 2(3):e174–e181.
12 Cauli M et al. *Dictionnaire francophone de la responsabilité sociale en santé*. Presses universitaires de Rouen et du Havre; 2019.

component of their social responsibility. Hence, our choice to design an African-based study was motivated by the need to consider the present concept of social responsibility in healthcare from this angle and by the lack of empirical studies on this issue. The aim was to evaluate the perceptions of patients and caregivers regarding the social responsibility of public hospitals.

Part I: Social responsibility in healthcare

Chapter 1: Corporate social responsibility

I. The concept of responsibility

1. What is responsibility?

Etymologically, the term « responsibility » is derived from « responsible » with the suffix -ity. It originates from the Latin verb « respondere » (« to be accountable »), akin to « spansio » (« promise »). This gives the word « responsibility » the meaning of « keeping one's promises ». The dictionary defines responsibility as follows: It is the obligation of the individual to be accountable for actions and roles they take upon themselves, burdens they should carry, and consequences they should bear thereof[13]. Thus, it stands for:

- The moral obligation or necessity to respond, to be accountable for one's actions and for those of others. E.g., She disclaimed all responsibility / liability for the accident.
- The case of being responsible for a specific function. E.g., He is responsible for the administration.
- A function or a position which gives decision-making powers, but for which one is accountable (especially in the plural form). E.g., They have responsibilities in the HR department.
- It also stands for something being the cause or the source of a damage. E.g., Responsibility of tobacco for lung cancer is a well-established fact.

2. Different types of responsibility

The different types of responsibility / liability include but are not limited to moral, public, civil, administrative, political, penal, and societal aspects.
Expressions including responsibility / liability are:

- **Civil liability insurance**: It is a contract which covers the insured against all pecuniary consequences of damage incurred to the public.

---

13 - Definition of responsibility. Dictionnaire français Larousse. Éditions Larousse; 2018.
   - Definition of « responsibility » – Centre national de ressources textuelles et lexicales (CNRTL) 2012. Available at: <https://www.cnrtl.fr/definition/responsabilité/>.
   - Definition of « responsibility ». Available at: <https://www.languefrancaise.com/dictionnaire/definition-responsabilite/>.
   - Dictionnaire de l'Académie française, 9e éd. Available at: <https://www.dictionnaire-academie.fr/article/A9R209>.

- **To take responsibility:** Acting on the ground that one can be held accountable for one's actions.
- **Civil liability:** is an obligation imposed by the law to repair the damage done to another either by the non-performance of a contract or by an intentional or nonintentional fault.
- **Collective liability**: is the act of imposing liability on a group whether the unlawful action is committed by a member of the group or by the whole group.
- **Public (or administrative) authority liability:** is a system which allows individuals to request compensation for the damage caused by the administration.
- **Vicarious liability**: is an obligation of one party to repair the damages that a third party has caused to others.
- **Governmental liability**: is a mechanism according to which the government may resign under the supervision of the parliament.
- **Medical liability**: is the doctor's obligation to avoid any damage to the patient or otherwise repair it.
- **Penal liability**: is an obligation to be accountable for one's actions and to perform the penal sanction prescribed for the criminal offence.
- **Moral responsibility**: is the necessity to be accountable for one's intentions and actions to one's conscience.
- **Political liability**: Jurists consider it as an advanced stage of accountability in a society where basic rights are being respected.
- **(Corporate) societal responsibility**: Also called social responsibility, it is the voluntary decision of businesses to consider the social and environmental concerns in their activities and interactions with other actors or "stakeholders".

II. Corporate social responsibility (CSR)

1. *Corporate social responsibility*

As an organisation situated at the heart of contemporary economic and social changes, the business is currently an «affair of society»[14]. The concept of corporate social responsibility (CSR) refers to a wider representation of the business's environment including not only in its economic and financial dimensions but also in its social, human, cultural, political, and economic ones. In this respect, CSR is at the centre of contemporary dynamics of capitalism and illustrates

---

14   Gond JP, Igalens J. *La responsabilité sociale de l'entreprise. Que sais-je?* 5e éd. France: PUF; 2016.

the capacity of this system to adapt to its critics by integrating them into its management mechanisms[15].

CSR also includes responsibility towards different interacting groups often referred to as stakeholders. In this light, as a business concept and practice, CSR remains ambiguous and complex. But contrary to some preconceptions, CSR is not a new concept; it rather stems from the extension of older corporate practices such as corporate philanthropy. It has been a topic of extensive academic discussion on the other side of the Atlantic since the 1920s[16].

2. *The foundations of CSR*

The concept of CSR is rooted in early American business practices spanning over a century during the Second Industrial Revolution, while its current resurgence in several European countries reflects a tradition of economic capitalism[17].

According to American historian Morell Heald, it is a conceptualisation of the relationship between the business and the community.

During the first two decades of the 20th century, the United States saw the emergence of a social reform environment dominated by progressive ideas and conducive to the development of this approach in business-society relations, giving rise to social responsibility. Economic collapse of the 1929 crisis and the decline in social prestige of leaders and businesses resulted in a reduction of discussions related to social responsibility[18]. It was not until the 1950s that CSR philosophy was reaffirmed again. Still, the development of CSR as an academic concept is quite recent coined by its "founding father" Howard R. Bowen. Published in 1953, his book *Social Responsibilities of the Businessman* represents one of the first systematic efforts to analyse the discourses and behaviours relative to social responsibility[19]. He defines CSR in this book as «obligations of businessmen to pursue those policies, to make those decisions, or to follow

---

15   Sainsaulieu R. *L'entreprise, une affaire de société*. Paris: Presses de sciences Po; 1992.
16   Heald M. *The social responsabilities of business. Company and community, 1900–1960*. Cleveland: Press of case western Reserve University; 1970; Pasquero J. La responsabilité sociale de l'entreprise comme objet des sciences de gestion: un regard historique » in M.-F. Bouthillier-Turcotte, A. Salmon, *Responsabilité sociale et environnementale de l'entreprise*. Sillery: Presses de l'Université du Québec; 2005, pp. 80–112.
17   Acquier A, Gond JP. Aux sources de la responsabilité sociale de l'entreprise: relecture et analyse d'un ouvrage fondateur: Social responsabilities of the businnessman d'Howard Bowen, 1953. *Finance-Contrôle- Stratégie* 2007; 10(2): 5–35.
18   Levitt T. The dangers of social responsibility. *Harvard Business Review* 1958; 36: 41–50.
19   Bowen HR. *Social responsibilities of the businessman*. New York: Harper; 1953.

those lines of conduct which are desirable in terms of the objectives and values of our society». It is, nevertheless, worth noting that Bowen's book, which marks the entry of CSR into the academic world, is part of a series of books devoted to the application of the Protestant doctrine to the lives of businessmen and to the economic problems of that era. This means that this definition of CSR initially had religious foundations and illustrated Marx Weber's thesis, showing affinities between Protestant ethics and the spirit of capitalism[20].

From this period on, CSR has been a subject of controversy around the political impacts of the company's involvement beyond economic prerogatives, thus becoming an "essentially contested" concept. In fact, CSR practices started to evolve in American corporations due to the influence of the social movements between 1960 and 1980[21].

3. CSR: Advocates vs. critics

Following the development of studies on CSR in the 1950s and 1960s, a new series of debates emerged in the context of the Cold War. On one side were the advocates of CSR who saw it as a selling point of the capitalist system to the American people. On the other side were critics who saw it as a real «Trojan horse» of communist ideology[22].

One of the first criticisms of CSR comes from Levitt who points to the potential political backlash. He invites business leaders to focus on the search for profit, acknowledge government and union involvement, and identify potential benefits[23].

In addition, as Friedman stipulates, business leaders who are not democratically elected have neither political legitimacy nor the required competencies for public service management.

---

20 Wood DJ. Corporate social performance revisited. *Academy of Management Review* 1991; 16(4): 691–718; Frederick WC, From CSR1 to CRS2: the maturing of business and society thought. working paper graduate school of business. Pittsburgh (PA), Pittsburgh Univ.; 1978.

21 Gond JP, Igalens J. *La responsabilité sociale de l'entreprise. Que sais-je?* 5e éd. France: PUF; 2016.

22 Acquier A, Gond JP. Aux sources de la responsabilité sociale de l'entreprise: relecture et analyse d'un ouvrage fondateur: Social responsabilities of the businnessman d'Howard Bowen, 1953, *Finance-Contrôle- Stratégie* 2007; 10(2): 5–35.

23 Levitt T. The dangers of social responsability. *Harvard Business Review* 1958; 36: 41–50.

4. The institutionalisation and theoretical foundations of CSR

Despite its deep roots in American and French contemporary history, CSR has only recently become a major concern for businesses. This is due to the initiative of international institutions, the emergence of new actors offering CSR innovative services, and the remarkable work of standardisation.

The European Commission published a Green Paper in 2001 entitled *Promoting a European framework for Corporate Social Responsibility*, which defines CSR as a concept whereby businesses "integrate social and environmental concerns in their business operations and in their interactions with their stakeholders on a voluntary basis". Two years earlier, in 1999, former United Nations (UN) Secretary-General Kofi Annan, expressed the international community's interest in CSR at the Davos Forum. He called upon the managers of large companies to join the Global Compact which comprises two principles of human rights, four principles on labour standards, three principles of environmental practices, and a principle of anti-corruption. Between 2008 and 2012, laws were passed in Europe and consultation platforms were established to bring together various stakeholders with an interest in CSR[24].

Standardisation in the field of CSR is increasingly important due to rising demand. Also, the regulatory bodies are showing a big interest in achieving success in CSR. ISO (International Standardisation Organisation) is the most prestigious body, a longstanding experience, and a recognised model through its ISO 9000 standard series. Besides, the ISO 26000 standard titled «guidance on social responsibility » was developed using a multi-stakeholder approach, with the participation of experts from 90 countries and 40 international organisations[25].

The research conducted by Bill Frederick and Donna Wood helps distinguish between three big stages of the theoretical development of CSR[26].

---

24   Gond JP, Igalens J. *La responsabilité sociale de l'entreprise. Que sais-je?* 5e éd. France: PUF; 2016.

25   Acquier A, Gond JP. Aux sources de la responsabilité sociale de l'entreprise: relecture et analyse d'un ouvrage fondateur: Social responsabilities of the businnessman d'Howard Bowen, 1953, *Finance-Contrôle- Stratégie* 2007; 10(2): 5–35.

26   Wood DJ. Corporate Social Performance revisited. *Academy of Management Review* 1991; 16(4): 691–718; Frederick WC. *From CSR1 to CRS2: the maturing of business and society thought. working paper graduate school of business.* Pittsburgh (PA), Pittsburgh Univ.; 1978.

- **The first period**, referring back to the 1950s and 1960s debates, was marked by a focus on the normative and philosophical aspects of CSR.
- **The second period**, between 1970 and 1980, witnessed the introduction of the notions of social responsiveness or sensitivityIn this period, emphasis was on corporate management of CSR process and the implementation of CSR practices.
- **The third period**, between 1980 and 2000, saw the emergence of a new concept replacing the notion of social sensitivity: It is *Corporate social performance (CSP)* which focussed onthe concrete results and impacts of CSR policies.

Additionally, as an interface of business and society, CSR allows for various definitions, theories, and approaches reflecting various representations of this business/society interface. Thus, CSR can be seen as:

- A social regulator (the functionalist approach) that seeks to align societal and corporate objectives;
- A power relationship (the socio-political approach) that seeks to answer the question: How can businesses dominate or be dominated by society?
- A cultural product (the culturalist approach) that considers how a business can adapt to its cultural environment;
- A socio-cognitive construct (the constructivist approach) that examines how the business and society can co-develop.

5. CSR: A stakeholder theory

The term « stakeholders » originated in the 1960s and gained wide popularity in the early 1980s following the works of Freeman[27]. A stakeholder is defined as any group or individual who directly or indirectly takes part in the activities of an organized system of actions, and who is positively or negatively affected by the achievement of the system's goals. In essence, it is any group or individual whose role is crucial for the survival and well-being of organisations or collaborations.

The stakeholder theory considers the interests and rights of all individuals and organizations that are cooperating with the business and are affected by various decisions. It emphasises the long-term role of stakeholders. Its importance for business ethics stems from its recognition of multiple values and from its nature as a moral act at different levels. Stakeholders are mainly affected by collaboration with an organisation and by its corporate activities. They, in turn, provide

---

27   Freeman RE. *Strategic management: a stakeholder approach*. Boston: Pitman; 1984.

guidance to the business in setting its goals and mission. Examples of stakeholders include the management, customers, shareholders, suppliers, and the broader society and community. This theory suggests that every organization or business seeks to make itself and its stakeholders successful. This means that maximising profit is not an issue in itself; it only becomes one if managers prioritise profit maximisation over activities that benefit key stakeholders, including society. By acknowledging reciprocity between businesses and stakeholders, Freeman challenges the idea that the main responsibility of business leaders is to maximize profits. He also invites these leaders to align the goals of their businesses with the interests of their stakeholders[28].

6. *Measuring CSR*

Measuring CSR is crucial for businesses to manage their social and environmental impacts. It can be realised through theoretical developments of corporate social performance (CSP)[29].

The main types of CSP measurements are as follows:

- Discourse measurement (This includes analysing the content of annual reports in words or themes related to CSR): This measurement not addressing the various dimensions of the construct is more symbolic than substantive;
- Pollution indicators: This measurement only focusses on the environmental aspect of the construct;
- Values and attitudes towards CSR: This involves questionnaire-based surveys;
- Indicators of reputation: This measurement can be mistaken for the notion of reputation. It can provide an overall measurement of CSP but has a degree of ambiguity;
- Auditing or measurement of processes, behaviours, or outcomes: This information is provided by measurement agencies.

It is worth noting that the tools commonly used in academia are those created by new CSR measurement practitioners from social and environmental rating agencies. Such measurements are somewhat objective because they are carried out by external organisations.

---

28 Siniora D. *Corporate social responsibility in the health care sector. 4th annual student symposium.* Dusquene Univ. Dusquene Scholarship collection; Aug. 25th. 2017.
29 Wood DJ. Corporate social performance revisited. *Academy of Management Review* 1991; 16(4): 691–718.

7. Financial impact of CSR

The financial impact of CSR allows for multiple theoretical explanations which can be categorised as follows[30,31]:

- The hypothesis that CSP has a positive influence on financial performance or positive social impact (meaning that greater inclusion of stakeholders leads to higher economic performance);
- The hypothesis that CSP has a negative influence on financial performance (indicating that investing in CSP increases costs and is therefore detrimental to financial performance;
- The hypothesis that financial performance has a positive impact on CSP, suggesting that the best economically performing businesses are also the best socially performing ones;
- The hypothesis that financial performance has a negative impact on CSP, . Also known as the hypothesis of managerial opportunism, it takes place when opportunistic managers strategically mobilize CSP investments to manipulate stakeholders;
- The hypothesis of positive, reciprocal impact between CSP and financial performance.

8. CSR economic and managerial implications

A survey[32] of a large number of executives from different nationalities found that most of them believed that CSR would be a high priority in the future. 52,9 % of them thought that CSR could help promote the image and reputation of their business. Additionally, for 53,3 % of these managers, CSR is a means of positioning and differentiation in the marketplace. These results indicate that economic motivation may underly CSR investments.

Finally, CSR presents theoretical and empirical contradictions. Although it is associated with globalisation, it is still relatively new to be in a globalised context. It remains a disputed concept which is likely to draw on different social movements depending on its environment.

---

30 Gond JP, Igalens J. *La responsabilité sociale de l'entreprise. Que sais-je?* 5e éd. France: PUF; 2016.
31 Waddock S. *The difference makers. How social and institutional entrepreneurs created the Corporate Responsibility Movement.* Sheffield: Greenleaf Publishing; 2008.
32 The 2007 Global Business Barometer. Economist Intelligence Unit. *The Economist* 2008.

III. Health-focussed corporate social responsibility (CSR)

1. CSR: Health investments

Regarding CSR, businesses generally invest in various sectors with a social impact on communities. Healthcare is a particularly significant area of investment in many countries, especially in Africa[33]. According to a 2013 survey funded by The United Nations Development Programme (UNDP) on the CSR practices of 100 Angolan businesses across different sectors, healthcare and education had received most of the budgetary allocations for CSR. The study also revealed that most Angolan businesses focussed on healthcare programmes for their employees and on HIV prevention in general[34,35].

Generally, health-focussed CSR investments can take the form of financial donations, humanitarian contributions, infrastructure reinforcement, and HR support (through financial backing for internships and healthcare professional training).

Apart from altruism and the humanitarian dimension, businesses get motivated by the outcomes generated by being engaged in promoting the health of their employees, families, and communities. In the context of globalisation, they are increasingly aware of the need for a triple-bottom-line (economic profit, social and environmental benefits). They invest not only human and financial resources but also in health programmes. What motivate them to support social and health programmes are:

– Cost savings: Healthy employees are more productive and have lower absenteeism. For example, one of the most inspiring stories of the impact of healthcare CSR on expenditure economy is the malaria programme implemented by South African gold mining giant AngloGold Ashanti in

---

33   A Review of Corporate Social Responsibility for Health in Africa. United States Agency for International Development; Dec. 2014. Available at: <http://www.africanstrategies4health.com/resources.aspx>.;
34   Business in development: AngloGold Ashanti and The Global Fund in Ghana. The United Kingdom Department for International Development (DFID) – Johns Hopkins Center for Communication Programs (CCP); 2017.
35   Shaping Corporate Social Responsibility in sub-Saharan Africa Guidance. Notes from a Mapping Survey. GIZ Center for Cooperation with Private Sector and University of Stellenbosch; 2013. Available at: <https://www.giz.de/expertise/downloads/giz2013-en-africa-csr-mapping.pdf>

Ghana[36]. In 2005, 6800 out of a total workforce of 8000 had malaria within one month; the cost for malaria treatment medication exceeded 55000 US dollars per month. The calculation of the costs associated with absenteeism and malaria treatment led the company to implement a comprehensive malaria control programme in the Obuasi community where the mining activity took place;
– Economic sustainability: a tangible example of health-focussed CSR for economic sustainability is cocoa cultivation in Africa. For instance, a chocolate factory made significant investments in CSR programmes to improve the quality of health, education, and agricultural services in Ghana and Ivory Coast which together contribute to 70 % of global cocoa production. This initiative helped prevent the shortage of this raw material required for chocolate production;
– Brand differentiation: Businesses that invest in health-focussed CSR may stand out from their competitors;
– Customer engagement: Businesses aim to build trust with their consumers and make them transaction partners by offering added-value services in support of social good;
– Employee engagement: Several studies have shown that employees who are more involved in CSR programmes are more engaged and more likely to remain in their workplace.

2. CSR approaches to healthcare

Businesses employ various approaches to carry out their CSR initiatives. This contributes to the betterment of health outcomes for employees, their families, their communities, and sometimes the general population. CSR engagement often focusses on maintaining employees' health and, by extension, the health of their families and communities[37].

For large businesses, this may also involve supporting a local clinic or providing in-house health services. The most common approaches include grants to NGOs

---

36   Business in development: AngloGold Ashanti and The Global Fund in Ghana. The United Kingdom Department for International Development (DFID) – Johns Hopkins Center for Communication Programs (CCP); 2017. Available at: <https://www.icmm.com/document/4673>.
37   A Review of Corporate Social Responsibility for Health in Africa. United States Agency for International Development; Dec. 2014. Available at: <http://www.africanstrategies4health.com/resources.aspx>.

or individuals, workplace health and wellness programmes, pro-bono expertise, or in-kind donations.

IV. Corporate social responsibility in healthcare

Healthcare providers have the same rights as individuals, and are treated like legal persons under the law. Just like individuals, they are moral agents and can be held morally responsible, meaning that they have both legal and moral obligations. Therefore, they have ethical obligations towards their societies, and are judged on how they treat their employees and carry out their missions[38,39].

Currently, the challenge for the healthcare sector, the government, medical profession, health care providers, and healthcare business managers is to promote the quality and equity of healthcare services through socially responsible activities. It is crucial then to fully embrace CSR and ethical principles to promote equal distribution of healthcare resources[40].

Healthcare organisations need to consider a wide range of health problems related to poverty around the world when integrating CSR. In the context of healthcare, social responsibility involves addressing issues related to human rights, gender equality, child labour, and the environment. The healthcare sector is expected to behave ethically and provide treatment for all individuals especially that it is under very significant pressure from policymakers, NGOs, media, and the public[41]. CSR activities should prioritise the most important health problems for more pertinence. In addition, Healthcare organisations and pharmaceutical industries are expected to be accountable to other stakeholders, society and future generations due to social and economic reality. Hence, the importance of CSR in the healthcare sector is well recognised, as it has been shown to lead to effective access to good medical practice[42].

---

38   Boelen C. *Défis et opportunités des partenariats pour le développement de la santé. Bases factuelles et information à l'appui des politiques Département de Prestation des services de santé*. WHO 2001.

39   Boelen C, Heck JE & World Health Organization. *Division of Development of Human Resources for Health. Définir et mesurer la responsabilité sociale des facultés de médecine / Charles Boelen et Jeffery E. Heck*. Genève: Organisation mondiale de la Santé; 2000. Available at: <https://apps.who.int/iris/handle/10665/66532>.

40   Siniora D. *Corporate social responsibility in the health care sector. 4th annual student symposium*. Dusquene Univ. Dusquene Scholarship collection; Aug. 25th. 2017.

41   Beauchamp TL, Childress JF. *Principles of biomedical ethics*. 7th ed. Oxford: Oxford University Press; 2013.

42   Brandão C, Rego G, Duarte I, et al. Social responsibility: A new paradigm of hospital governance?. *Health Care Analysis* 2013; 21(4): 390–402.

1. Social responsibility in healthcare: The role of healthcare organisations and pharmaceutical industries

Healthcare organisations and pharmaceutical companies have a mission to contribute to the common good and to create various types of added value to society. With their integrated ethical values, knowledge and resources, they should focus their CSR activities on addressing health problems and enhancing people's quality of life. These activities can take various forms, such as[43]:

- A socially responsible hospital or pharmaceutical industry should find the best ways to treat or carefully dispose of a waste product that might be environmentally hazardous.
- Pharmaceutical industries can improve the patients' quality of life and reduce costly hospitalisations by researching, thereby serving a significant social interest.

In this context, it should be noted that CSR requires combined efforts of individual stakeholders, governments, donors, NGOs, and the private sector to act in terms of skills, techniques, knowledge and strengths of each party. Furthermore, the CSR of these organisations depends on their willingness to cooperate with other parties. CSR in healthcare differs from CSR in other industries because medicine and medical care services are essential to human well-being. The fact that the poor cannot buy costly medicines because of the market requirements, patents, and the absence of generic medicines or affordable substitutes for patented ones is an outrageous reality for both society and the international community[44]. Hence, several programmes run by the healthcare sector were proposed to provide affordable access to medicines for the poor. For example, the twenty largest pharmaceutical industries have taken strong CSR-based initiatives, and the majority of them have developed basic CSR teams. Thus, social responsibility in healthcare should respond to the stakeholders' demands, the goals of the healthcare facilities and the universal ethics requirements in order to help alleviate human suffering and improve the lives of individuals and communities. However, a successful integration of the strategies of social responsibility into day-to-day practice takes time and effort from healthcare managers.

---

43 Brewer KM. Corporate social responsibility in the pharmaceutical industry – why it matters from business, bioethical and social perspectives (Thesis). Winston- Salem (NC): WAKE FOREST Univ., 2014.
44 Collins SK. Corporate social responsibility and the Future Health Care Manager. *The Health Care Manager* 2010; 29(4): 339–345.

2. Social responsibility and health governance

The 2014 report from USAID (United States Agency for International Development) defines governance as "a collective process of decision making for ensuring vitality and performance of healthcare organisations"; "it fixes the strategy and goals, elaborates policies, laws, rules, regulations, and decisions; it mobilises and deploys resources needed to achieve this strategy and goals, and it supervises and ensures that they are implemented"[45]. Health governance aims to protect and promote the health of individuals and populations while also meeting society's needs. Therefore, managers should demonstrate a clear commitment to improve the performance of healthcare systems through social responsibility. According to several field studies (USAID, 2014), there are five governance practices:

a. Performance optimisation to improve service provision.
b. Stakeholder engagement.
c. Development of a common strategic direction.
d. Optimal resource management.
e. Governance assessment for further improvement.

3. Social responsibility in healthcare: The role of healthcare managers and leaders

Healthcare organisations are currently facing new challenges, emphasising the need for effective management skills and proper stakeholder engagement. Research has shown that organisations with enlightened managers who prioritise CSR in their daily practice are better equipped to meet public expectations. The implementation of CSR is closely linked to the values and beliefs of the managers, as they establish ethical standards for their businesses[46]. In healthcare organisations, inaccuracies in management plans and misjudgements of managers can have serious consequences for all stakeholders. Therefore, it is crucial for healthcare managers to receive ethical training within their professional roles, and to seek ethical advice to fulfil their missions. This underscores the importance of accountability in healthcare management.

---

45 Cauli M, Boelen C, Ladner J. et al. *Dictionnaire francophone de la responsabilité sociale en santé*. Presses universitaires de Rouen et du Havre; 2019.
46 Frunză S. Ethical responsibility and social responsibility of organizations involved in the public health system. *Revista de cercetare și intervenție socială* 2011; 32: 155–171.

Chapter 2: Values and obligations of healthcare organisations

1. Values of social responsibility in healthcare

Social responsibility in healthcare is based on the values of quality of care provision, equitable access to healthcare services, and the pertinence and efficiency of allocated resources[47] (figure 1).

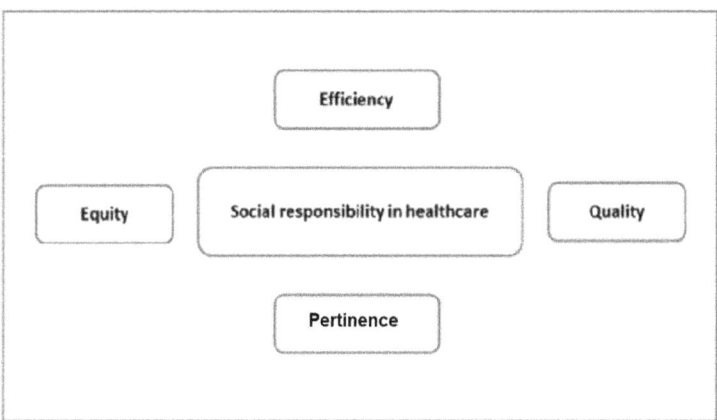

Figure 1: The values of social responsibility in healthcare

(a) **Quality:** The quality of healthcare holds great importance. The main guiding principle and point of reference for a population's health is to improve the health of its individuals. In this respect, quality can be defined as the capacity to provide responses to individual health problems. The concept of health quality involves not only caregivers but also patients. It varies according to the socio-economic status as well as the availability of qualified staff.

(b) **Equity:** "Health for All" is a major goal of WHO, focussing on the value of equity to reduce all forms of discrimination based on race, sex, religious

---

47 Boelen C, Heck JE & World Health Organization. *Division of Development of Human Resources for Health. Définir et mesurer la responsabilité sociale des facultés de médecine / Charles Boelen et Jeffery E. Heck.* Genève: Organisation mondiale de la Santé; 2000. Available at: <https://apps.who.int/iris/handle/10665/66532>

beliefs, ethnic affiliation, socio-economic status, or age. It also aims to establish health policies that allow all individuals to access healthcare services, enjoy a fulfilling life, and easily obtain information about risk factors for disease. Promoting awareness of equity in health covers the entire population, including vulnerable subgroups that face exclusion from essential health services.

However, it is challenging to prioritise both quality and equity in healthcare due to the high costs and limited budgets. Some patients can benefit from technology-based health solutions, while others struggle to access even basic health services. Balancing quality and equity is still possible by considering two additional values: pertinence and efficiency.

(c) **Pertinence:** It measures how well the choices and priorities of action programmes align with the most significant health problems, which is not an easy task. The criteria of pertinence change regularly based on epidemiological data. Thus, the principle of pertinence can ensure both quality and equity while the healthcare system remains primarily focussed on disadvantaged subgroups. However, "rationalisation" or the choice of priority areas should be justified, as it may sometimes be seen as a reduction of health services and could lead to controversies.

(d) **Efficiency:** Tt refers to the ability to utilise available resources for service delivery by comparing the benefits of therapeutic interventions with other options. In some cases, preventive measures may be considered more cost-effective than curative care.

To conclude, health care organisations, pharmaceutical industries, and medical schools should prioritise four values of social responsibility: quality, equity, efficiency, and pertinence, and consider the need to effectively integrate them into their operations. This approach will enable managers and leaders of healthcare systems to develop customised action plans that address individual and collective needs.

2. The ethics of healthcare organisations

Ethics is an old concept that originated from moral philosophy. It encompasses both theoretical manifestations, such as philosophical debates, or practical manifestations that focus on the moral validation of human actions. In the context of health, ethics calls upon states, organisations, and individuals to make sound decisions in extreme situations of healthcare inequalities with longevity gaps in order to ensure access to quality care. The ethics of healthcare organisations comprises three interrelated but distinct areas[48,49]:

- The organisation's moral dimension is expressed in its mission and values. The head of the health organisation is then expected to embody the role of the ethics officer.
- The capacity to identify and solve ethical challenges.
- The integration of organisation ethics into the management process.

Adhering to ethics programmes and their regulatory and legal requirements help organisations minimise the risk of severe penalties. These programmes are therefore mandatory and are endorsed by the administration. Organisations that uphold ethical principles should have a set of values suitable for health promotion and patient care, and should know how to address complex situations in healthcare.

An organisation's ethics is demonstrated in its endeavours to find the best possible solutions for problems in accordance with predefined values. In this context, the scarcity of resources in the healthcare sector compels organisations to act in a way that is both ethically justifiable and clinically valid[50].

In their book entitled *Social Justice*, Madison Powers and Ruth Faden explain the ethical reasons why all human beings have a right to well-being. They argue that well-being involves six irreducible dimensions: health, personal security, developing and utilising cognitive capacities for reasoning, living under conditions of social respect, developing and maintaining deep personal connections, and being able to lead a self-determining life. They recommend that governments, NGOs, and businesses should collectively take responsibility for these aspects[51].

Pharmaceutical businesses develop new therapies to alleviate suffering while still generating profits. Nonetheless, Powers and Faden contend that for businesses to be morally ethical, they should facilitate access to medication for the world's poor. This can be achieved in many ways, such as developing cures for

---

48 Kashyap R et al. Corporate social responsibility: a call for multidisciplinary inquiry. *Journal of Business & Economics Research* 2004; 2(7): 51–58.
49 Magill G, Prybil L. Stewardship and integrity in health care: a role for organizational ethics. *Journal of Business Ethics* 2004; 50(3):225–238.
50 Spencer E et al. *Organization ethics in health care*. Oxford: Oxford University Press; 2000.
51 Powers M et Faden R. *Social justice: The moral Foundations of Public Health and Health Policy (Issues in biomedical ethics)*. New York: Oxford University Press; 2006.

overlooked tropical diseases, providing free medication for poor communities, donating to deprived areas, creating low-cost facilities for essential medicines, and issuing transitional medication certificates to foreign industries for the development of certain medicines. It is important to note that the healthcare sector alone cannot address the root causes of poverty. This is because the burden of the social dimension of human health conditions falls more on international economic organisations, including the World Bank, the International Monetary Fund (IMF), and international governments operating under an international economic structure. Therefore, collaboration between pharmaceutical companies and hospitals on one side, and governments, international institutions and NGOs on the other, can help achieve social and healthcare equity[52,53,54,55].

3. Social responsibility in healthcare: A moral obligation

Article 14 of the UNESCO International Bioethics Commission report on social responsibility in healthcare refers to this concept as part of a new standard of hospital governance. This standard requires hospitals and other healthcare organisations achieve their goals in light of rights and general ethical standards. The report suggests that social responsibility should be viewed as a moral obligation to create organisational value. What sets this article apart is its broader application of the concept of social responsibility, extending not only to the private sector but also to the public and governmental sectors, with the aim of acknowledging and providing healthcare as a universal right based on universal principles.

UNESCO's first Director General, Julian Huxley, believes that in order for science to contribute to peace, security and human well-being, it is essential to align the uses of science and values. This highlights the importance of social responsibility in healthcare, which aims to reshape decision-making in bioethics

---

52   Lee M, Kohler J. Benchmarking and transparency: incentives for the pharmaceutical industry's corporate social responsibility. *Journal of Business Ethics* 2010; 95(4): 641–658.
53   Leisinger KM. The Corporate social responsibility of the pharmaceutical industry: idealism without illusion and realism without resignation. *Business Ethics Quarterly* 2005; 15(4): 577–594.
54   Oger C. *Corporate social responsibility in the pharmaceutical industry: between trend and necessity*. Library and Archives Canada; 2010.
55   Takahashi T et al. Corporate Social Responsibility and hospitals: US theory, Japanese experiences, and lessons for other countries. *Healthcare Management* 2013; 26(4): 176–179.

and address vital concerns of many countries. Advances in science and technology should improve access to quality healthcare, essential medication, nutrition, and water. These advances should also be linked with improvements in living conditions, environmental quality, and reduction in poverty and illiteracy rates. Despite the development of new medications and technologies, global healthcare issues still persist. In this context, actions driven by social responsibility could significantly help reduce reducing healthcare inequalities, uphold human rights, and foster social capital[56,57,58].

---

56   Brandão C, Rego G, Duarte I, et al. Social responsibility: a new paradigm of hospital governance?. *Health Care Analysis* 2013; 21(4): 390–402.
57   Siniora D. *Corporate social responsibility in the health care sector. 4th annual student symposium.* Dusquene Univ. Dusquene Scholarship collection; Aug. 25th. 2017.
58   Martinez-Palomo A. *The UNESCO Universal Declaration on bioethics and human rights. Background, principles and application.* Paris: UNESCO Publishing; 2009.

Chapter 3: The ethical principles of social responsibility in healthcare

1. The principle of justice

Article 25 of the UN Declaration on Human Rights states that "everyone has the right to a standard of living adequate for the health and well-being of himself and of his family, including food, clothing, housing and medical care and necessary social services, and the right to security in the event of unemployment, sickness, disability, widowhood, old age or other lack of livelihood in circumstances beyond his control". Therefore, social justice includes the human right to health, based on the idea that health and access to medication should be a universal human right. Pharmaceutical industries and healthcare organisations have a moral responsibility to provide access to medication for disadvantaged people while achieving their sustainable business objectives[59,60]. According to John Rawls' principle of justice, equity is essential to justice in healthcare. This means that everyone, regardless of their social status, should have equal access to healthcare services[61].

2. The principle of beneficence

Pharmaceutical industries and health organisations have an obligation to respect the principle of beneficence in addition to the principle of justice. In their *Principles of Biomedical Ethics*, Beauchamp and Childress describe beneficence as more than just kindness or charity; it is also as an obligation to help others and further their interests. It is important to note that beneficence is assumed to be integrated into all medical professions, health education and vaccination programmes. Healthcare organisations have a moral responsibility to conduct research on medicines that can help people in deprived areas, meaning that the interests and values of all stakeholders should be taken into account.

---

59 Siniora D. *Corporate social responsibility in the health care sector. 4th annual student symposium.* Dusquene Univ. Dusquene Scholarship collection; Aug. 25th. 2017.
60 Brewer KM. Corporate social responsibility in the pharmaceutical industry – why it matters from business, bioethical and social perspectives (Thesis). Winston- Salem (NC): WAKE FOREST Univ., 2014.
61 Beauchamp TL, Childress JF. *Principles of biomedical ethics.* 7th ed. Oxford: Oxford University Press; 2013.

Chapter 4: The social responsibility of faculties of medicine

1. Social responsibility in healthcare: The role of faculties of medicine

Faculties of medicine are currently challenged to have a more significant impact on people's health and to demonstrate this with concrete results. This emphasises the concept of social responsibility, which was officially defined by the WHO in 1995 as the obligation of faculties of medicine to meet the priority health needs of their communities[62]. In recent decades, medical training has focussed on technical competence and specialisation. Although this focus resulted in qualified doctors, it was more doctor-centred than patient or community-centred. Social responsibility aligns with the scientific approach of evidence-based medicine, as it involves a commitment to achieving results through training, research, service provision, and to verifying their impacts on patients, the public and, society in general[63].

Cultivating social responsibility requires the commitment of faculties of medicine to ensure that educational programmes are responsive to people's needs. Additionally, training should extend beyond teaching hospitals to community-based ambulatory care practices where most healthcare is delivered. These experiences will influence the future career choices and practices of medical students[64]. However, identifying healthcare needs, helping medical students acquire the necessary skills, and addressing under-medicalised areas require joint efforts from policymakers, faculties of medicine, health-service managers, doctors, and patients. In theory, faculties of medicine could be better placed to promote coordination between market analysis, product formation

---

62 Meili R, Buchman S. La responsabilité sociale: au cœur de la médecine familiale. *Canadian Family Physician* 2013; 59(4): 344–345.
63 Boelen C. Consensus Mondial sur la Responsabilité Sociale des Facultés de Médecine. *Santé publique* 2011; 23(3): 247–250.
64 Boelen C, Interlinking medical practice and medical education. Prospects for international action. In: Walton H, ed., Proceedings of the world summit on medical education. Medical Education, 1994; suppl. 1, 28: 82–85.

and distribution. In practical terms, production -or training per se- is often the main focus[65].

The decision to incorporate social responsibility into the curriculum of faculties of medicine led to the development of numerous programmes. However, the main challenge lies in implementing these programmes due to the slow response of medical training structures to change. In 2009, an international reference group of 130 representatives, including leading associations of faculties of medicine and worldwide organisations of medical education, engaged in substantive reflection and exchange around social responsibility of faculties of medicine. This effort resulted in the unanimous adoption of a document entitled "Global Consensus on Social Accountability of Medical Schools" which highlights the need to enhance the faculty's capacity to address the health needs and challenges of individuals and society, in line with the values of social responsibility in healthcare, namely quality, equity, pertinence and efficiency.

---

65   Boelen C. Consensus Mondial sur la Responsabilité Sociale des Facultés de Médecine. *Santé publique* 2011; 23(3): 247–250.

Chapter 5: The social determinants of health

Health problems are largely attributed to the social conditions in which people live and work. All over the world, disadvantaged people have less access to health resources, are more susceptible to disease, and have a lower life expectancy compared to privileged people[66,67]. Nowadays, healthcare services are increasingly seen as a fundamental right, but people's health is affected by the paradox of scientific progress. On the one hand, this progress has led the development of new medicines, surgical techniques, and increasingly effective diagnostic tools, thereby improving people's life expectancy and quality of life. However, the world health situation is inequitable due to poverty and the lack of access to healthcare.

1. What are the social determinants of health?

The social determinants of health are interconnected social, political, economic, and cultural factors that shape the circumstances in which people are born, grow, live, and age. These factors evolve and change over time, impacting the health of individuals and communities in different ways. As per the WHO Commission on Social Determinants of Health (2008), these determinants encompass social, physical, and economic environments, as well as individual characteristics and behaviours. People's health is influenced not only by their living environments, but also by their genetic makeup, personal choices, and lifestyles.

Key determinants influencing health include[68]:

- Income and social status: Individuals with a higher income and a privileged social status tend to have better health.
- Education (literary and health knowledge): Lower educational levels are associated with poor health, increased stress, and lower self-confidence.
- Physical environment: Access to safe water, clear air, healthy workplaces, secure housing, safe communities and roads, non-exposure to violence, and availability of transportation all contribute to good health.

---

66 Walker RJ, Smalls BL, Campbell JA et al. Impact of social determinants of health on outcomes for type 2 diabetes: a systematic review. *Endocrine* 2014 Sept; 47(1): 29–48.
67 Lucyk K, McLaren L. Taking stock of the social determinants of health: a scoping review. *PLoS ONE* 2017; 12(5): e0177306.
68 Walker RJ, Smalls BL, Campbell JA et al. Impact of social determinants of health on outcomes for type 2 diabetes: a systematic review. *Endocrine* 2014 Sept; 47(1): 29–48.

- Employment and working conditions: Employed individuals, particularly those with more control over their working conditions, tend to be healthier than the unemployed.
- Social support networks, discrimination, or social inclusion: Strong support from families, friends, and communities is linked to better health.
- Culture: Family and community customs, traditions, and beliefs impact health;
- Genetics: Inheritance plays a role in determining lifespan, health, and susceptibility to certain illnesses.
- Personal behaviour and coping skills: Balanced eating, physical activity, smoking, alcohol consumption, and stress management all affect health.
- Health services: Accessibility and use of healthcare services influence people's health.
- Gender: Men and women experience different health issues at different ages.

The list of social determinants continues to expand to include new parameters. In addition to the classic determinants, such as nutrition, education and access to health, other determinants have been identified, including:

- Race and racism
- The ethnic background
- Native ancestry, colonisation, and the migratory experience

This means that the health policy encompasses not only the provision and financing of medical care, but also the lifelong impact of health determinants in early childhood, as well as the effects of poverty, unemployment, malnutrition, working conditions, drug use, social supports, and lifestyle issues such as access to adequate food social status[69].

As a result, the WHO Commission on the Social Determinants of Health outlined the following overarching recommendations: (a) to improve the conditions of daily life– the circumstances in which people are born, grow, live, work, and age; (b) to address the unequal distribution of power, money and resources – the structural drivers of those conditions of daily life – globally, nationally and locally; (c) to measure the problem, evaluate action, develop a workforce that is trained in the social determinants of health, and raise public awareness about the social determinants of health.

---

[69] Walker RJ, Smalls BL, Campbell JA et al. Impact of social determinants of health on outcomes for type 2 diabetes: a systematic review. *Endocrine* 2014 Sept; 47(1): 29–48.

2. The social determinants of health: An ambiguous concept

The term "social determinants of health" can be confusing for several reasons. Firstly, there is no consensus on the criteria or taxonomy that define what should be considered a social determinant of health. The term "social" is ambiguous and difficult to define precisely. Additionally, the extensive list of determinants may discourage healthcare practitioners from actively seeking them out and referring patients to support services when needed. It is also important to consider how much emphasis should be placed on each determinant, which determinants should be prioritised, and the basis for such prioritisation. The lack of clarity and the continually expanding list of determinants are the main reasons for the variability characterising the social determinants of health in the literature. Furthermore, the confusion may lead to the presumption that policies focussing only on the social determinants of health can reduce health inequalities, which is a simplistic explanation of the whole concept[70]. Moreover, the concept of "social determinants of health" can be misleading as it refers, according to Graham[71], to both the determinants of health and the determinants of health inequalities. For this reason, it was suggested that the concept should be replaced by a more precise one, such as "social determinants of health inequities". Finally, all existing ambiguities and confusions should be eliminated to ensure a clear understanding of the concept for all relevant stakeholders, including the public, for better results in health and well-being.

3. Actions related to the social determinants of health

It is important to address the social determinants of health to alleviate the burden of disease and promote good health for the entire population. The problems are especially urgent in developing countries where the burden of chronic diseases is added to that of infectious ones[72].

Several initiatives are being taken in different parts of the world to address health inequalities[73]. These measures are meant to reduce inequalities in the

---

70 Islam MM. Social Determinants of Health and Related Inequalities: confusion and implications. *Frontiers in Public Health* 2019; 7: 11.
71 Powers M., Faden R. Social justice: The moral foundations of public health and health policy (Issues in biomedical ethics). New York: Oxford University Press; 2006.
72 Walker RJ, Smalls BL, Campbell JA et al. Impact of social determinants of health on outcomes for type 2 diabetes: a systematic review. *Endocrine* 2014 Sept; 47(1): 29–48.
73 Lucyk K, McLaren L. Taking stock of the social determinants of health: a scoping review. *PLoS ONE* 2017; 12(5): e0177306.

global health situation and to improve health for all by meeting the health needs of disadvantaged populations. One South American initiative consisted of creating a commission on the social determinants of health. Another initiative, based on European studies, is centred on addressing inequalities in people' access to healthcare by improving educational opportunities, income distribution, and hygiene behaviour. A third initiative, concerned with knowledge networks to identify opportunities for improved action in key areas, emphasised the vital role of national governments and civil society in achieving greater health equity[74].

---

74 Islam MM. Social determinants of health and related inequalities: confusion and implications. *Frontiers in Public Health* 2019; 7: 11.

Part II: The situation of health in Africa

Chapter 1: The context and situation of health in Africa

I. The African continent

Africa is a vast continent, covering 6 % of the Earth's surface and 20 % of the global land surface. It stretches 8,000 km from north to south and 7,500 km from west to east, covering an area of 30 million Km² with 22,500 km of coastline, which is three times the size of Europe. Africa is bordered by the Mediterranean Sea to the north and the Atlantic Ocean to the west. It is divided into two hemispheres by the equator, and connected to Asia through the Suez Canal and the Red Sea to the north-east, and is quite close to Europe through the Strait of Gibraltar[75,76]. The inhospitable coasts and shores have been more of a hinderance than an opening, and poor internal infrastructures and communication networks have long isolated the continent.

The continent is characterised by droughts, and is known as the hottest continent in the world. It has remarkably diverse natural areas, including plains, valleys, plateaus, and mountains[77]. Sixty percent of the land is arid, and its environment is particularly rich with the second largest continuous forest massif on the planet. However, deforestation and decline in biodiversity, as consequences of climate change and human pressure, are putting this environment in danger[78,79,80]. Africa, being the cradle of humankind, is nowadays under-populated due to slave trade, disease, malnutrition, and war. Weakened largely by colonial exploitation, African economy is based on farming, stockbreeding, and handicraft.

---

75 Pitte JR. Atlas de l'Afrique, Les éditions du Jaguar; 2011.
76 Monot T, Afrique (Structure et milieu). Biogéographie, Encyclopædia Universalis. Éditeur Primento; 2016.
77 Pak Sum Low. *Climate change and Africa*. Cambridge University Press; 2006.
78 Hugon P. L'Afrique: Défis, enjeux et perspectives en 40 fiches pour comprendre l'actualité. Eyrolles éditions; 2016. Available at: <https://www.eyrolles.com/Chapitres/9782212564846/9782212564846.pdf>
79 Tout l'univers- Encyclopédie. Le livre de Paris-Hachette. Paris: Hachette Collections SNC; 2014.
80 Pulley Sayre A. Africa. Twenty-First Century Books; 1999.

The African continent can be divided into two major regions[81,82,83]

- **Northern Africa,** also known as "white Africa" or "the Maghreb", borders black Africa. Its vast deserts are adjacent to forest areas. This region needs to address the challenge of high demographic growth rates, modernising its economy, and developing its healthcare systems.
- **Central and Southern Africa,** located south of the equator, is characterised by vast open spaces, decimated wildlife, and politically instable countries periodically shaken by conflicts and civil wars.

Africa is frequently divided into five regions (figure 2):

- **North Africa,** bounded to the south by the Sahara, is inhabited by populations mostly of Arab and Berber origins, including **Morocco, Algeria, Tunisia, Libya, Egypt, and Sudan.**
- **Sub-Saharan Africa,** which is divided into four sub-regions:

- *West Africa*: Benin, Burkina Faso, Cape Verde, Ivory Coast, Gambia, Ghana, Guinea, Guinea Bissau, Mauritania, Liberia, Mali, Niger, Nigeria, Senegal, Sierra Leone, and Togo.
- *East Africa*: Burundi, Comoros, Djibouti, Eritrea, Ethiopia, Kenya, Madagascar, Malawi, Mauritius, Rwanda, Seychelles, Somalia, Somaliland, Tanzania, South Sudan, Uganda, Zimbabwe, and Zambia.
- *Central Africa*: Angola, Cameroon, Chad, Central African Republic, Republic of Congo, Democratic Republic of Congo, Equatorial Guinea, Gabon, and Sao Tome and Principe.
- *Southern Africa*: Located in the south of the equatorial forest, it includes **Mozambique, Lesotho, Botswana, Namibia, South Africa, and Eswatini.**

---

81 Tout l'univers- Encyclopédie. Le livre de Paris-Hachette. Paris: Hachette Collections SNC; 2014.
82 Drysdale A, Blake GH. *The Middle East and North Africa*. USA: Oxford University Press; 1985.
83 Composition des régions macrogéographiques (continentales), composantes géographiques des régions et composition de groupements sélectionnés économiques et d'autres groupements. [archive]. Organisation des Nations unies; 2015.

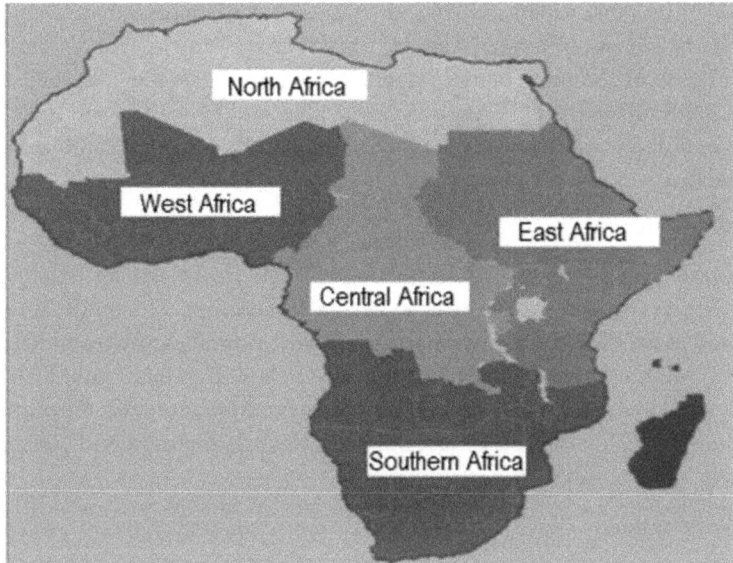

Figure 2: African regions

1.1 African demographics

The population of Africa nearly tripled from approximately 478 million in 1980 to around 1.2 billion in 2015. It is expected to reach 1.5 billion by 2025 and around 2.4 billion by 2050. The annual rate of population growth increased to 2.5 % from 1980 to 2015 and is projected to remain at 1.5 % in the next ten years. Sixty-one percent of the total population growth in the continent over the 1980–2015 period was represented by ten countries: Nigeria, Ethiopia, the Democratic Republic of Congo, Egypt, the United Republic of Tanzania, Kenya, Uganda, Sudan, South Africa, and Algeria[84].

– Demographic distribution

Africa is the least urbanised continent in the world, despite rapid urbanisation. The current urban population is estimated to be at 40 %, compared to only 27 %

---

84 Profil démographique de l'Afrique. Addis-Abeba (Éthiopie): Commission économique des Nations Unies pour l'Afrique; Mar. 2018. Groupe de la publication et de l'impression de la CEA, certifié ISO 14001:2004.

in 1980[85]. The most urbanised African countries are Gabon, Libya, Democratic Republic of Congo, Djibouti, Algeria, Cape Verde, Tunisia, Congo, and South Africa. Some of the most densely populated countries in the continent are the Island States of Mauritius, Comoros, Seychelles, and Sao Tome and Principe, as well as mainland countries such as Rwanda, Burundi, Nigeria, Gambia, Uganda, and Malawi.

– Total fertility rate

The average fertility rate in African regions has decreased by half over the past thirty years, and this trend is expected to continue. Currently, the rate is estimated at 4.7 children per woman, but it varies significantly from country to country. Some countries like Mauritius, Seychelles, Tunisia, South Africa, and Algeria have low rates, while others such as Niger, Mali, Somalia, Chad, Angola, the Democratic Republic of Congo, Burundi, Uganda, Gambia, and Nigeria have relatively higher rates[86,87,88,89].

– Early pregnancy

Adolescent pregnancy (aged 15–19) is still prevalent in Africa, with the highest rates recorded in Niger (40.4 %) and Mozambique (37.5 %) as well as in Chad, Central African Republic, Guinea, Congo, Madagascar, and Nigeria. In contrast,

---

85   CEA, Commission de l'Union africaine et FNUAP: « Déclaration d'Addis-Abeba sur la population et le développement après 2014 ». Addis-Abeba (Éthiopie); 2013. Available at: <www.unfpa.org/sites/de-fault/les/event-pdf/declaration- nal-e1351225.pdf>.
86   Profil démographique de l'Afrique. Addis-Abeba (Éthiopie): Commission économique des Nations Unies pour l'Afrique; Mar. 2018. Groupe de la publication et de l'impression de la CEA, certifié ISO 14001:2004.
87   CEA, Commission de l'Union africaine et FNUAP: « Déclaration d'Addis-Abeba sur la population et le développement après 2014 ». Addis-Abeba (Éthiopie); 2013. Available at: <www.unfpa.org/sites/de-fault/ les/event-pdf/declaration- nal-e1351225.pdf>.
88   CEA, Union africaine, Groupe de la Banque africaine de développement et Programme des Nations Unies pour le développement: Rapport sur les OMD 2014: Évaluation des progrès accomplis en Afrique dans la réalisation des objectifs du Millénaire pour le développement. Addis–Abeba; 2014. Available at: <www.uneca.org/sites/default/les/PublicationFiles/2014_mdg_report.pdf>.
89   Division de la population de l'ONU: Perspectives de la population mondiale: Révision de 2015. New York: United nations; 2015. Available at: <http://esa.un.org/unpd/wpp/>

these pregnancies are relatively fewer in the North African sub-region, especially in Tunisia (2.9 %)[90].

– Infant and child mortality

Despite Africa's significant efforts to reduce infant mortality, the progress remains insufficient. For instance, the infant mortality rate declined to less than 100 deaths per 1000 births in all African countries over the period 2010–2015. The highest rates in the continent were recorded in Angola, Chad, and Sierra Leone. Additionally, the mortality rate for children under five is higher in South Sudan, Mali, Sierra Leone, Angola, Guinea Bissau, Chad, Somalia, Nigeria, Burundi, and the Central African Republic[91,92].

– Maternal mortality

In the period between 1990 and 2015, Africa successfully reduced its maternal mortality rate by half. The countries that saw a decline in mortality declined include Sierra Leone, the Central African Republic, Chad, Nigeria, South Sudan, Somalia, Liberia, Burundi, Gambia, and the Democratic Republic of Congo[93,94,95].

---

90 Division de la population de l'ONU: World Urbanization Prospects: The 2014 Revision. New York: United nations; 2014. Available at: <https://www.un.org/en/development/desa/publications/2014-revision-world-urbanization-prospects.html>
91 Integrating Population Issues into Sustainable Development, including the post-2015 Development Agenda: a concise report: publication des Nations Unies. United nations; 2015. Available at: <www.un.org/en/development/desa/population/commission/pdf/48/CPD48ConciseReport.pdf>.
92 OMS, UNICEF, FNUAP, Groupe de la Banque mondiale et Division de la population des Nations Unies, Tendances de la mortalité maternelle: 1990–2015. Genève: Organisation mondiale de la santé; 2015. Available at à l'adresse:
    <http://apps.who.int/iris/bitstream/10665/194254/1/9789241565141_eng.pdf>.
93 Profil démographique de l'Afrique. Addis-Abeba (Éthiopie): Commission économique des Nations Unies pour l'Afrique; Mar. 2018. Groupe de la publication et de l'impression de la CEA, certifié ISO 14001:2004.
94 CEA, Union africaine, Groupe de la Banque africaine de développement et Programme des Nations Unies pour le développement: Rapport sur les OMD 2014: Évaluation des progrès accomplis en Afrique dans la réalisation des objectifs du Millénaire pour le développement. Addis–Abeba; 2014. Available at: <www.uneca.org/sites/default/les/PublicationFiles/2014_mdg_report.pdf>.
95 OMS, UNICEF, FNUAP, Groupe de la Banque mondiale et Division de la population des Nations Unies, Tendances de la mortalité maternelle: 1990–2015. Genève: Organisation mondiale de la santé; 2015. Disponible à l'adresse:
    <http://apps.who.int/iris/bitstream/10665/194254/1/9789241565141_eng.pdf>.

– Life expectancy

From 1980 to 2015, life expectancy at birth in Africa increased from 50 years to almost 60 years by 2010–2015. This positive trend is expected to continue, reaching 70 years by 2050. Eritrea, Ethiopia, Algeria, Morocco, and Niger had the highest life expectancy rates during the 1980–2015 period. However, life expectancy in other countries such as Swaziland, Lesotho, Zimbabwe, the Ivory Coast, and South Africa decreased over the same period, mainly because of HIV and AIDS.

– Age structure of the population

The population of Africa is predominantly young. Children aged 0–14 make up about two-fifths of the population, and those aged 15–24. Children aged 0–14 make up nearly one-fifth. In 1980, children aged 0–14 represented almost 45 % of the African population. By 2015, this age group accounted for 473.7 million people. The population aged 25–64 grew faster than other age groups, increasing from 123.7 million (33.3 %) in 1980 to 425.7 million (36.2 %) in 2015. In addition, the number of older people (aged 65 and above) increased from about 15 million in 1980 to over 40 million in 2015. However, this age group remains the smallest of the total population, representing 3.1 % in 1980 and 3.5 % in 2015.

– Net migration

The number of migrants in Africa is low compared to other parts of the world. In 2015, Africa's net migration (the difference between immigration into and emigration from an area in a given period) decreased by 2.9 million in 2015, and it is expected to drop to 2.3 million by 2050. It is important to note that African countries serve as countries of origin, transit, and destination for migrants. The most common type of migration in the region is labour migration, followed by forced migration, illegal migration, and transit migration[96,97].

---

96 Profil démographique de l'Afrique. Addis-Abeba (Éthiopie): Commission économique des Nations Unies pour l'Afrique; Mar. 2018. Groupe de la publication et de l'impression de la CEA, certifié ISO 14001:2004.

97 Mitra S, Posarac A, Vick B. Disability and poverty in developing countries: a snapshot from the World Health Survey". Social protection and labor. The World Bank. 2011; pp. 33–34.

1.2 The African society

The African society is built on extended family and ethnic background. There are around a thousand ethnic groups across the continent, forming the basis of solidarity and community cohesion. Africa has also about 2000 living spoken languages, making it the most linguistically diverse region in the world[98,99].

However, the African population faces challenges in formal education. Primary school enrolment rates in Sub-Saharan Africa dropped to 71 % in 1990, with significant differences between countries. North Africa has much higher enrolment rates[100]. As for higher education, UNESCO reported in 2012 that student enrolment in higher education institutions in Sub-Saharan countries increased by about twenty-five times compared to 1970. This increase is due to population growth and efforts by various states to improve access to primary and secondary education. Despite this, the continent has the lowest tertiary enrolment rates at 6 % according to UNESCO, compared to 13 % in South and West Asia, and 72 % in North America and Western Europe[101,102]. The continent also faces economic challenges, with 47 % of the African population living below the poverty line of less than 1.25 US dollars PPP per day. Despite this, urbanisation has led to the growth of a significant middle class, willing to participate in cultural and economic globalisation, as well as striving for democracy and good governance[103].

1.3 The African economy

Even though poverty is decreasing, there continues to be a rise in the proportion of poor people in Africa, indicating that the decrease is slower compared to other parts of the world. The continent's economy and exports are largely based

---

98   Chrétien JP, Le défi de l'ethnisme. Rwanda et Burundi: 1990 – 1996 (fiche bibliographique du centre de documentation du CNRS). Paris: éd. Karthala; 1997.
99   Chrétien JP, Mukuri M. Burundi, la fracture identitaire: logiques de violence et certitudes ethniques, 1993–1996, Paris: éd. Karthala; 2002.
100 D'Almeida-Topor H. L'Afrique du xxe siècle à nos jours. éd. Armand Colin. coll. « U »; 2013.
101 D'Almeida-Topor H. L'Afrique du xxe siècle à nos jours. éd. Armand Colin. coll. « U »; 2013.
102 Caramel L. Éducation: l'Afrique toujours dans le peloton de queue. Le Monde 9 avr. 2015.
103 Jacquemot P. Les classes moyennes changent-elles la donne en Afrique? Réalités, enjeux et perspectives. *Afrique contemporaine* 2012; 244: 17–31.

on extractive industries, with Africa being rich in oil and possessing 30 % of the world's mineral reserves. Africa also has a significant amount of available farmland, which is of interest to countries like the Gulf, India, and China. About 5 % of the continent's land is owned by foreign countries through purchase or lease[104,105,106]. It is worth noting that the continent's position in world trade is currently weak, accounting for around 3 % in value, and only 1.6 % of world GDP. In addition, the 1980s and 1990s were marked by a debt crisis in Africa. But the early 21st century witnessed a decrease in the debt burden although the debt levels are still being closely monitored [107].

– The infrastructures

Africa faces a significant infrastructure deficit, particularly in the areas of electricity and transportation. Investing in infrastructure is essential for economic growth, businesses, and the well-being of the population. This is because it enables access to water, to which 65% of African populations are connected, and to electricity, to which only 29% of Africans have access[108].

– Governance

According to Transparency International, Africa is considered to be one of the continents where corruption is most widespread. Since 2007, the index assessing the effectiveness of public action in the African states has established a classification based on a score system ranging from 1 to 100. The continent's average score showed a slight increase from 49.9 in 2007 to 50.1 in 2016. The highest regional average was recorded in Southern Africa at 58.9, while the lowest score was recorded in Central Africa at 40.9[109,110]. Overall, Eastern and

---

104 La diversification économique: une urgence pour l'Afrique. Afrique renouveau. Nations Unies; avr. 2011. p. 26.
105 Kuikeu, O. Conséquences de l'instabilité politique de l'Afrique: la trappe de la dépendance à l'égard des matières premières » [archive]. Atelier des médias, RFI, 12 juill. 2012.
106 *Afrique subsaharienne. Un changement de cap s'impose.* coll. « Perspectives économiques régionales », Fond monétaire international ; avr. 2016.
107 Brunel S. L'Afrique est-elle si bien partie? éd. sciences humaines; Oct. 2014.
108 Lumenganeso O. L'Afrique doit d'abord investir dans ses infrastructures. Les Afriques; 31 août 2010.
109 Essoungou AM. La bonne gouvernance, clé du progrès. Afrique Renouveau; août 2010.
110 Perspectives économiques en Afrique – Gouvernance politique et économique en Afrique. 2016; 5: 131.

Southern Africa, as well as the coastal countries of West Africa, are demonstrating remarkable dynamism, while the regions of the Sahel, Central Africa, and the Horn of Africa are prey to conflict and remain rentier economies.

- Informal economy

The informal economy in Africa makes up between 40 % and 75 % of the GDP, significantly impacting the continent's economy. Around 66 % of job opportunities in Sub-Saharan Africa are in the informal sector, yet the tax burden remains low and insufficient. At the macroeconomic level, the informal economy serves as a means of social and economic resilience in response to growth that does not adequately create jobs[111,112].

- Natural resources

Africa heavily depends on raw materials, which account for 60 % of its exports. However, the continent lacks local industry to add value to these natural resources. Agriculture has tripled its value since the 1980s, due to expanded food production areas, but this has come at the expense of forests and the savannah. Despite this growth, African agriculture suffers from low productivity, lack of irrigation and mechanisation, and small farmland size. In 2006, agricultural products represented 20 % of Africa's international trade and 30 % of the value of its exports[113]. Despite having the second largest the number of fishing boats in the world after Asia), Africa's fleet is the least equipped globally. Morocco stands out as the only African country, ranking 17th out of 25 countries, with 82 % of global fisheries[114,115].

- Services

The services sector in African countries is steadily growing, and now accounts for more than 50 % of their GDP. This growth is mainly due to exports,

---

111   Berrou JP, Gondard-Delcroix C. Dynamique des réseaux sociaux et résilience socio-économique des micro-entrepreneurs informels en milieu urbain africain. Mondes en développement 2011; 4(156): 73–88.
112   Alderson K, Meale E. Industries extractives – Vue d'ensemble [archive]. Banque mondiale; 15 Sept. 2015.
113   Appauvrissement et dégradation des terres et des eaux: menace grandissante pour la sécurité alimentaire. FAO; 28 Nov. 2011.
114   Guinée: la pêche industrielle interdite pendant deux mois [archive]. RFI; 2 juill. 2016.
115   Polle B. Afrique de l'Ouest: les rouages de la pêche illégale passés au crible. Jeune Afrique 29 jui. 2016.

including agricultural products[116]. as well as domestic consumption driven by population growth. Even with limited infrastructure, there is a strong demand for telecommunication services. From 2009 to 2012, the services sector made up 32.4 % of total employment in Africa, largely due to informal employment in small businesses, particularly in commerce, catering, and transport. On the global scale, Africa contributes 2.2 % to total exports of services and 4 % to total imports, but its competitiveness is hindered by unfavourable regulations and poor infrastructure[117].

– Macroeconomic performance in Africa

In 2018, economic growth in Africa was estimated at 3.5 %, marking a 1.4 % increase from the 2.1 % recorded in 2016. There were variations in growth rates across regions. Despite the positive prospects for growth, there are risks associated with increased tensions in global trade and uncertainties surrounding commodity prices[118].

– Employment, growth, and business dynamism in Africa

The working-age population in Africa is expected to increase by around 40 % by 2030. However, it is projected that only 50 % of the job seekers will find employment, and many of these opportunities will be in the informal sector, leading to a high rate of youth unemployment. Despite rapid economic growth over the past two decades, there has been limited job creation.

The main challenges to industrialisation in Africa include inadequate infrastructure, limited business growth, and an unsupportive regulatory environment for business development. According to corporate surveys conducted by the World Bank, between 1.3 and 3 million jobs are lost annually due to corruption, inadequate infrastructure, and bureaucracy. Additionally, small and medium-sized businesses have limited opportunities to expand in most African countries.

---

116 Rapport sur la compétitivité en Afrique 2015: Transformer les économies africaines [archive]. Banque mondiale; 2015.
117 Perspectives économiques en Afrique 2011. OECD, African Development Bank, United Nations Economic Commission for Africa. United Nations Development Programme; 2011
118 Perspectives économiques en Afrique 2019. Groupe de la banque africaine de développement; 2019

II. The situation of health in Africa

The African continent is known for its diversity, with differences in culture, economy, politics, and governance among countries. So, it is impractical to use a single approach to address the health situation in all these countries. Since 2000, Africa has experienced economic growth, leading to a dramatic decrease in poverty. Investments targeting urgent health needs have contributed to the improvement of health and well-being of the African populations. Still, it is important to acknowledge the challenges in meeting their health needs. The health situation in the African region can be analysed from the following dimensions[119]:

– The healthy life expectancy of individuals and communities
– The causes of morbidity and mortality
– The risk factors of morbidity and mortality
– Healthy life expectancy in Africa

The concept of healthy life expectancy refers to the number of years that a person is expected to live in good health. This measures provides valuable insights compared to overall life expectancy alone, as it indicates the difference between merely being alive and living in a state of good health or poor health. In the African Region, healthy life expectancy rose from 50.9 to 53.8 years between 2012 and 2015, marking the most significant increase among all WHO regions. However, disparities between countries persist, with the longest healthy lifespans typically found in economically well-off countries with better economies while improvement is occurring more rapidly in countries with large populations and high population density. Despite progress, the levels of healthy life in the African Region still lag significantly behind other parts of the world[120].

– The major causes of morbidity and mortality in Africa

The main causes of morbidity and mortality in Africa include communicable diseases, non-communicable diseases (NCDs) such as cardiovascular and kidney

---

119 État de la santé dans la région africaine de l'OMS: Analyse de la situation sanitaire, des services et des systèmes de santé dans le contexte des objectifs de développement durable. Organisation mondiale de la Santé, Bureau régional de l'Afrique; 2018.
120 Statistiques sanitaires mondiales 2017: Suivi de la santé pour les ODD. Organisation mondiale de la santé; 2017.

diseases, violence, and traumas. Lower respiratory tract diseases, HIV/AIDS, and diarrhoeal diseases remain significant contributors to morbidity and mortality. However, it is important to note that the rates of morbidity and mortality have decreased considerably due to fewer cases of malaria, HIV/AIDS, and diarrhoeal diseases. The overall death rate from these primary causes has also dropped from 87.7 to 51.3 per 100.000 people, although there has not been a notable reduction in the rate of non-communicative diseases[121].

– The risk factors of morbidity and mortality in Africa

It is crucial to consider the risk factors that contribute to health morbidity and mortality. According to the WHO, the fight against NCDs (chronic respiratory diseases, cardiovascular diseases, cancer, and diabetes) relies on addressing four risk factors: physical inactivity, smoking, alcohol abuse, and poor diet). Currently, an African aged between 30 and 70 has a 20.7 % chance of dying from one of these major NCDs. The lowest probability of dying from these diseases was recorded in regions with access to high-quality, specialised healthcare services.

Physical inactivity and poor diet are more common among women, while smoking is more prevalent among men. Certain risk factors, particularly smoking, disproportionately affect women, especially adolescent girls. Despite improvements in healthy living and reductions in morbidity and mortality, current levels in Africa remain lower than in other parts of the world. Additionally, the heavy burden of risk factors does not guarantee well-being and quality of life[122,123].

III. The health situation of African populations

Access to healthcare services is crucial for people's health regardless of their needs or location. Only 48 % of the expected healthcare services are delivered in Africa,

---

121 État de la santé dans la région africaine de l'OMS: analyse de la situation sanitaire, des services et des systèmes de santé dans le contexte des objectifs de développement durable. Organisation mondiale de la Santé, Bureau régional de l'Afrique; 2018.
122 État de la santé dans la région africaine de l'OMS: Analyse de la situation sanitaire, des services et des systèmes de santé dans le contexte des objectifs de développement durable. Organisation mondiale de la Santé, Bureau régional de l'Afrique; 2018.
123 Statistiques sanitaires mondiales 2017: Suivi de la santé pour les ODD. Organisation mondiale de la santé; 2017.

with significant variation between different African countries. A country's health index tends to improve as its gross domestic product (GDP) increases, indicating a strong correlation between a country's income and the health of its population[124,125,126].

– Availability of essential services

The availability of essential services reflects the availability of healthcare supply. It is crucial that these services meet the needs of the population. At only 0.36, the overall score for essential services availability in Africa is extremely low. This means that, on average, countries in this region provide their populations with just 36 % of the essential services needed for maintaining health and well-being. Adolescents and elderly people are the most affected age groups by the shortage of essential service. Additionally, healthcare systems in Africa tend to focus only on a small number of "priority services" (Table 1).

---

124 État de la santé dans la région africaine de l'OMS: Analyse de la situation sanitaire, des services et des systèmes de santé dans le contexte des objectifs de développement durable. Organisation mondiale de la Santé, Bureau régional de l'Afrique; 2018.

125 Rapport sur la santé dans le monde, 2000 – Pour un système de santé plus performant, Genève: Organisation mondiale de la Santé; 2000. Available at: <http://www.who.int/iris/handle/10665/42281>

126 Atlas des statistiques sanitaires africaines 2016. Analyse de la situation sanitaire de la Région africaine. Observatoire africain de la santé, Organisation mondiale de la Santé, Bureau régional de l'Afrique OMS (2017), Financement de l'acc ès universel à l'eau, l'assainissement et l'hygiène dans le cadre des objectifs de développement durable. Rapport d'analyse et d'évaluations globales de l'assainissement et de l'eau potable (GLAAS) 2017 de l'ONU-Eau. Genève: Organisation mondiale de la Santé; 2017.

Table 1: Key reference services for each age cohort[127]

Pregnancy and new-borns	Childhood	Adolescence	Adulthood	Old age
• Prenatal care • Perinatal care • Postnatal care	• Childhood vaccination • Childhood nutrition (malnutrition & overnutrition) • Integrated child services • Primary school care • Promotion of a healthy lifestyle for children	• Adolescent Sexual and reproductive care. • Adolescent- and youth-friendly care. • Secondary school care. • Anti-drug & anti-alcohol prevention. • Promotion of a healthy lifestyle for adolescents.	• Testing for common communicable diseases. • Testing for common non-communicable diseases and associated risk factors. • Reproductive care, including family planning. • Promotion of a healthy lifestyle for adults. • Nutrition services for adults. • Clinical and recovery care.	• Annual check-up and medical examinations. • Social support services for the elderly. • Clinical and recovery care for the elderly.

Source: Ne laisser personne de côté: Renforcement des systèmes de santé pour la CSU et les ODD en Afrique. Brazzaville: Bureau régional de l'OMS de l'Afrique, 2017

– Coverage of essential health interventions

Essential health interventions should be available across all public health functions, including health promotion, prevention of communicable and non-communicable diseases, and curative, rehabilitative, or palliative care. However, standing at only 0.57, the index for essential health interventions is low, indicating that people in the African Region are only benefiting from 57 % of these interventions. While communicable disease control received the highest score of 0.76 compared to other public health functions, a quarter of the population still does not receive treatment for these diseases. On the other hand,

---

127 État de la santé dans la région africaine de l'OMS: analyse de la situation sanitaire, des services et des systèmes de santé dans le contexte des objectifs de développement durable. Organisation mondiale de la Santé, Bureau régional de l'Afrique; 2018.

non-communicable diseases (NCDs) control scored the lowest at 0.44, reflecting very low access to treatment for these diseases despite the high burden of NCDs in the African Region[128]. Furthermore, there are significant inequalities in the use of health services in the region[129]:

- The higher a country is ranked economically, the better its essential medical interventions score is;
- Countries with higher healthcare expenditure have better access to services, especially curative and rehabilitative ones;
- Inequalities in access to interventions exist not only between countries, but also within each country;
- Financial risk protection levels also vary.

Financial risk protection aims to lower the barriers that prevent communities from accessing essential services by reducing the operating costs for households and individuals. Out-of-pocket payments are a major barrier to accessing essential services when there are insufficient funds[130,131,132]. The financial risk protection index varies by country, ranging from 0.1 to 0.7 out of 1. With a

---

128 Atlas des statistiques sanitaires africaines 2016. Analyse de la situation sanitaire de la Région africaine. Observatoire africain de la santé, Organisation mondiale de la Santé, Bureau régional de l'Afrique OMS (2017), Financement de l'acc ès universel à l'eau, l'assainissement et l'hygiène dans le cadre des objectifs de développement durable. Rapport d'analyse et d'évaluations globales de l'assainissement et de l'eau potable (GLAAS) 2017 de l'ONU-Eau. Genève: Organisation mondiale de la Santé; 2017.
129 Rapport sur la santé dans le monde, 2000 – Pour un système de santé plus performant, Genève: Organisation mondiale de la Santé; 2000. Available at: <http://www.who.int/iris/handle/10665/42281>
130 État de la santé dans la région africaine de l'OMS: analyse de la situation sanitaire, des services et des systèmes de santé dans le contexte des objectifs de développement durable. Organisation mondiale de la Santé, Bureau régional de l'Afrique; 2018.
131 Rapport sur la santé dans le monde, 2000 – Pour un système de santé plus performant, Genève: Organisation mondiale de la Santé; 2000. Available at: <http://www.who.int/iris/handle/10665/42281>
132 Atlas des statistiques sanitaires africaines 2016. Analyse de la situation sanitaire de la Région africaine. Observatoire africain de la santé, Organisation mondiale de la Santé, Bureau régional de l'Afrique OMS (2017), Financement de l'acc ès universel à l'eau, l'assainissement et l'hygiène dans le cadre des objectifs de développement durable. Rapport d'analyse et d'évaluations globales de l'assainissement et de l'eau potable (GLAAS) 2017 de l'ONU-Eau. Genève: Organisation mondiale de la Santé; 2017.

score of 0.34, it indicates that only 34 % of the maximum protection possible is provided in the region. This level of financial risk protection index is mainly due to low government investment in social security; it is also influenced by a country's income, as higher income correlates with a higher index[133].

– The levels of appropriate health security

Africa is particularly vulnerable to epidemics, making it crucial to identify and monitor at-risk populations in order to address their needs. Health security is achieved when a country has the basic capacity to prevent, detect, and respond effectively to health-related disasters[134].

In the African region, countries have only 57 % of the required skills, the lowest rate among all WHO regions. Furthermore, there are disparities in health security status among countries, with a clear correlation between score and income level. High-income countries have the highest scores. Ultimately, health security measures are more reliable in wealthy countries compared to poorer ones regardless of the area of focus[135].

– Responsiveness of essential services to people's needs

Ensuring that essential services responsive to people's needs is a crucial goal for any healthcare system. The factors used to measure responsiveness include autonomy, dignity, confidentiality, timeliness of care, access to social support, quality infrastructure, and choice of healthcare providers.

---

133 Atlas des statistiques sanitaires africaines 2016. Analyse de la situation sanitaire de la Région africaine. Observatoire africain de la santé, Organisation mondiale de la Santé, Bureau régional de l'Afrique OMS (2017), Financement de l'acc ès universel à l'eau, l'assainissement et l'hygiène dans le cadre des objectifs de développement durable. Rapport d'analyse et d'évaluations globales de l'assainissement et de l'eau potable (GLAAS) 2017 de l'ONU-Eau. Genève: Organisation mondiale de la Santé; 2017.

134 Rapport sur la santé dans le monde, 2000 – Pour un système de santé plus performant, Genève: Organisation mondiale de la Santé; 2000. Available at: <http://www.who.int/iris/handle/10665/42281>

135 Atlas des statistiques sanitaires africaines 2016. Analyse de la situation sanitaire de la Région africaine. Observatoire africain de la santé, Organisation mondiale de la Santé, Bureau régional de l'Afrique OMS (2017), Financement de l'acc ès universel à l'eau, l'assainissement et l'hygiène dans le cadre des objectifs de développement durable. Rapport d'analyse et d'évaluations globales de l'assainissement et de l'eau potable (GLAAS) 2017 de l'ONU-Eau. Genève: Organisation mondiale de la Santé; 2017.

Key participants shared their perspectives on the responsiveness of their healthcare system. The results, showing the proportion of positive responses for each factor, were calculated based on the responses received. The responsiveness index was then determined by averaging these results. The index value (0.47) is primarily linked to access to social support (0.73), autonomy (0.37), and quality of facilities (0.27), all of which are the areas with the lowest levels of responsiveness.

IV. Healthcare systems in Africa

During the first decades after gaining independence, most healthcare systems in Africa were built on the colonial health model. Large hospitals played a vital role in providing healthcare to urban populations. In addition, the battle against the major endemic diseases relied heavily on financial support from external public or private funding, particularly through specialised programmes targeting diseases like AIDS or malaria[136].

– An organisation chart

Healthcare systems and practices in Africa are supported by the UN health organisations such as WHO, UNICEF, and UNFPA[137]. The healthcare systems follow a pyramid model (figure 3):

- First-level structures that deal with common pathologies, community care, and maternal health are the primary care dispensaries and health huts.
- District or regional hospitals with 50 to 200 beds provide out-patient consultations and hospitalisation services for medicine, paediatrics, surgery, maternity, and sometimes emergency care. They are part of the national healthcare system, consisting of hospitals and medical centres serving an area with 100,000 to 200,000 inhabitants. This is also where essential health information tools for collecting epidemiological data are installed[138].

---

136   Jacquemot P. Les systèmes de santé en Afrique et l'inégalité face aux soins. *Afrique contemporaine* 2012; 3(243): 95–97.
137   De la Moussaye E, Jacquemot P. Politique de santé, les trois options stratégiques. *Afrique contemporaine* 1993; 166: 15–26.
138   Görgen H, Kirsch-Woik T, Schmidt-Ehry R. Le Système de santé de district. Expériences et perspectives en Afrique. Manuel à l'intention des professionnels de santé publique. 2e éd. Wersbaden, GTZ; 2004.

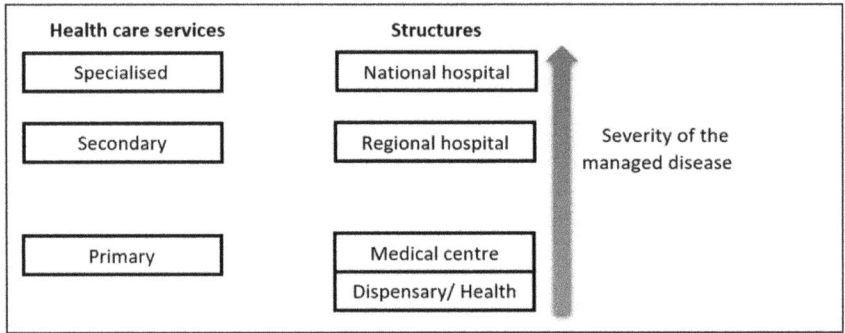

Figure 3: A sample of the African healthcare system[139]

– The healthcare sector

Primary-level hospitals provide care for common pathologies, maternal and child health, and community-based care. They may also perform minor surgeries. District hospitals have one bed for every 1,000 inhabitants. In rural areas, there is one medical centre/dispensary for every 6,000 inhabitants, and in urban areas, there is one for every 10,000 inhabitants. The nearest medical centre/dispensary should be no more than 5 km away (or 10 km in hard-to-reach areas)[140].

In terms of staffing, a 200-bed hospital should have at least three doctors, one nurse for every three beds, an administrator/manager, and two specialised hospital technicians. A dispensary should have a head nurse, a midwife, a nursing assistant or a social worker. As for the district management team, it should include a public health doctor as chief doctor, a senior staff nurse, a hospital manager, a maternal and childcare manager, and an accountant, among others[141].

– Healthcare provision

Effective coordination among different stakeholders at different levels is crucial for ensuring good patient care. In Africa, healthcare can be provided by public, private or faith-based organisations, while quality and outcome control

---

139 Jacquemot P. Les systèmes de santé en Afrique et l'inégalité face aux soins. *Afrique contemporaine* 2012: 3(243): 95–97.
140 Görgen H, Kirsch-Woik T, Schmidt-Ehry R. Le Système de santé de district. Expériences et perspectives en Afrique. Manuel à l'intention des professionnels de santé publique. 2e éd. Wersbaden, GTZ; 2004.
141 Jacquemot P. Les systèmes de santé en Afrique et l'inégalité face aux soins. *Afrique contemporaine* 2012: 3(243); 95–97.

are generally overseen by the public sector. The number of private healthcare providers and traditional practitioners is increasing. Additionally, a significant number of public healthcare providers also operate in the private sector. As a result, while healthcare practice is theoretically regulated, it often lacks real control[142].

It is important to acknowledge the significant contribution of faith-based or charitable organisations to the healthcare systems of countries where they are located. In Africa, nearly half of the total healthcare expenditure is incurred in the private sector. This varies depending on the specific political and economic circumstances of each country. For example, in countries like Uganda and Ghana, the private sector accounts for more than 60 % of healthcare expenditure, while in others like Namibia, it is less than 10 %. Approximately two-thirds of private sector healthcare activity is commercially driven while the remainder is charitable. This formal healthcare sector includes faith-based institutions, NGOs, pharmacies, manufacturers, and importers. On the other side, there is an informal health sector that consists of traditional healers, practitioners, and street vendors who cater mainly to underserved, rural populations by offering non-approved medicinal products[143].

– Inequal access to healthcare

The distribution of public health expenditure tends to favour wealthy urban dwellers over the rural poor. For example, in Mauritania, 72 % of hospital subsidies go to the richest 40 % of the population. In Ghana, 33.3 % of health expenditure benefits the richest segment, compared to only 12 % for the poorest. This inequality is due to the high cost of specialised healthcare and educational facilities, which are typically located in high-income urban areas[144].

It is important to identify priorities and set objectives in healthcare policy in times of limited resources[145]. This involves determining funding sources for the healthcare system (such as taxes or health insurance), as well as allocating resources between preventive and curative actions for effective health planning.

---

142 Investir dans la santé en Afrique. Le secteur privé: un partenaire pour améliorer les conditions de vie des populations. Washington: Groupe de la Banque mondiale; 2008.
143 Investir dans la santé en Afrique. Le secteur privé: un partenaire pour améliorer les conditions de vie des populations. Washington: Groupe de la Banque mondiale; 2008.
144 De la Moussaye E, Jacquemot P. Politique de santé, les trois options stratégiques. *Afrique contemporaine* 1993: 166: 15–26.
145 Van Lerberghe W, De Brouwere V. État de santé et santé de l'État en Afrique subsaharienne. *Afrique contemporaine* 2000; 195: 175–190.

V. The performance of healthcare systems in Africa

The effectiveness of a healthcare system is determined by its ability to provide necessary health services to the population based on their needs. The WHO assesses system performance according to four dimensions: access to essential services, quality of essential services, effective demand for essential services at the community level, and the system resilience to withstand shocks[146,147].

In Africa, the average system performance index is 0.49, indicating that African healthcare systems operate at only 49 % of their potential functionality. Besides, the performance indexes in African countries range from 0.26 to 0.70. All dimensions of system performance are under-performing, with the lowest performance seen in system resilience and access to essential services (figure 4).

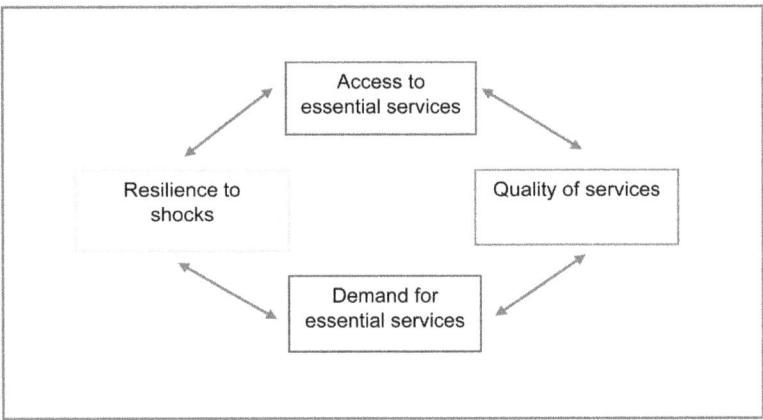

Figure 4: The characteristics of healthcare system performance

– Access to essential services

The African region has poor access to essential healthcare services, with an access index of 0.32, meaning that, on average, only 32 % of essential services are

---

146 État de la santé dans la région africaine de l'OMS: analyse de la situation sanitaire, des services et des systèmes de santé dans le contexte des objectifs de développement durable. Organisation mondiale de la Santé, Bureau régional de l'Afrique; 2018.
147 Health system strategy. WHO; 2007. Available at: <http://www.who.int/healthsystems/strategy/en/>

accessible. This is due to inadequate infrastructure, staff, and products in African countries[148].

- The quality of essential health services

The quality-of-care index for healthcare in the African region is 0.63, indicating that the quality of care is only 63 % of what is possible. This index varies widely between countries in the region, ranging from 0.25 to 0.94. In order to improve quality, it is important to consider the population's perception and the effectiveness of interventions[149].

- The demand for health services at the community level

This reflects the potential of households and communities to utilise essential healthcare services. In the African region, the demand score is relatively high compared to other performance measures, and its variation across countries does not appear to be dependent on income levels. This score indicates that healthcare systems are delivering the services people need. However, more progress can be achieved since the actual demand score of 67 % is still low and does not meet the required performance level[150,151].

- The resilience of health systems

System resilience prevents essential services from being disrupted by shocks. In the African region, system resilience levels are low, directly contributing to the frequent and devastating impact of epidemics and disasters. The region's

---

148 État de la santé dans la région africaine de l'OMS: analyse de la situation sanitaire, des services et des systèmes de santé dans le contexte des objectifs de développement durable. Organisation mondiale de la Santé, Bureau régional de l'Afrique; 2018.
149 Atlas des statistiques sanitaires africaines 2016. Analyse de la situation sanitaire de la Région africaine. Observatoire africain de la santé, Organisation mondiale de la Santé, Bureau régional de l'Afrique OMS (2017), Financement de l'accès universel à l'eau, l'assainissement et l'hygiène dans le cadre des objectifs de développement durable. Rapport d'analyse et d'évaluations globales de l'assainissement et de l'eau potable (GLAAS) 2017 de l'ONU-Eau. Genève: Organisation mondiale de la Santé; 2017.
150 État de la santé dans la région africaine de l'OMS: analyse de la situation sanitaire, des services et des systèmes de santé dans le contexte des objectifs de développement durable. Organisation mondiale de la Santé, Bureau régional de l'Afrique; 2018.
151 Health system strategy. WHO; 2007. Available at: <http://www.who.int/healthsystems/strategy/en/>

resilience levels are only at 39 % of what is needed to ensure the delivery of essential services during epidemics and disasters.

VI. The situation of investments in healthcare systems

To achieve universal health coverage, countries should invest in seven key areas: health workforce, health infrastructure, health products, service provision, health governance, health financing, and health information.

On average, 60 % of healthcare expenditure in African countries is on tangible investments (health workers, health infrastructure and health products) at the expense of intangible investments. Within tangible investments, the highest spending is on health products (39 % of public expenditure), followed by healthcare staff (14 %), and then infrastructure (only 7 %). A high-performing healthcare system allocates more resources to healthcare staff (40 % vs. 14 %) and infrastructure (33 % vs. 7 %)[152][153] (figure 5).

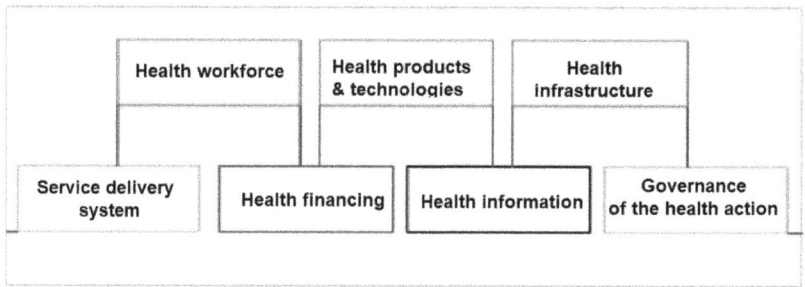

Figure 5: A ranking of healthcare system investment areas

– The situation of the health workforce in Africa

The health workforce is an essential component of healthcare systems, and should be adequate, skilled, and well-managed. The scores for the health workforce vary widely from country to country, ranging from 0.74 to 0.02, revealing big differences in the region. The most available staff are nurses, followed

---

152 État de la santé dans la région africaine de l'OMS: analyse de la situation sanitaire, des services et des systèmes de santé dans le contexte des objectifs de développement durable. Organisation mondiale de la Santé, Bureau régional de l'Afrique; 2018.

153 Observatoire mondial de la santé de l'OMS. OMS; 2020. Available at: <https://www.who.int/gho/database/fr/>

by community health workers and health management staff. Additionally, it is important to note that high-income countries invest more in the healthcare workforce[154].

- The situation of the health infrastructure in Africa

Evaluating the health infrastructure situation is based on health infrastructure scores. This should take into account several factors such as the availability, functioning, and readiness of different types of infrastructure[155,156]. However, the information available in all countries of the region is related to:

- The overall readiness of structures to provide essential services (availability of electricity, water, and other services for service delivery);
- The presence of basic equipment and materials required for service delivery;
- The overall density of hospitals, health centres, and hospital beds (per 100,000 inhabitants).

In Africa, the scores vary widely across countries, ranging from 0.06 to 0.67. But this overall score is insufficient to achieve the desired system performance.

- The situation of health products in Africa

Health products, such as medicines, vaccines, traditional remedies, medical devices, diagnostic tools, laboratory equipment, and blood products, are essential components of healthcare services. Ensuring the availability and quality of these products is crucial for the delivery of effective healthcare. The scores for available and quality health products vary widely between African countries, ranging from 0.87 to 0.1. The majority of countries in the region have scores between 0.4 to 0.55, indicating a consistent situation of health products in many African countries [157].

- The situation of the service delivery system in the African region

---

154 État de la santé dans la région africaine de l'OMS: analyse de la situation sanitaire, des services et des systèmes de santé dans le contexte des objectifs de développement durable. Organisation mondiale de la Santé, Bureau régional de l'Afrique; 2018.
155 Health system strategy. WHO; 2007. Available at: <http://www.who.int/healthsystems/strategy/en/>
156 Observatoire mondial de la santé de l'OMS. OMS; 2020. Available at: <https://www.who.int/gho/database/fr/>
157 État de la santé dans la région africaine de l'OMS: analyse de la situation sanitaire, des services et des systèmes de santé dans le contexte des objectifs de développement durable. Organisation mondiale de la Santé, Bureau régional de l'Afrique; 2018.

Service delivery includes all actions that are necessary to facilitate the effective management of inputs for service delivery. In Africa, there are shortfalls in the design, funding and monitoring of health service delivery systems. As a result, the use of available resources is hardly effective[158].

– The situation of health governance systems in the African region

The performance of health service is strongly influenced by the governance systems in place. Governance is made up of various interconnected attributes. To evaluate its quality, key informants from the region were requested to share their views on governance issues in their countries. A substantial percentage of informants (51 %) believed that national health officials lacked stability in guiding policy implementation, thereby constraining the capacity for health governance in the region[159] (figure 6).

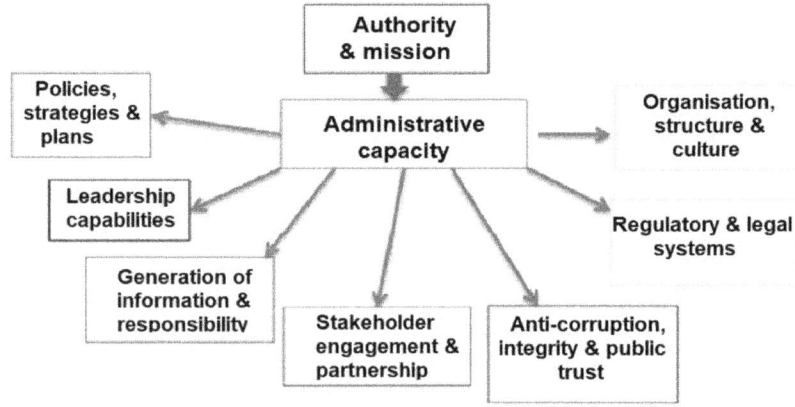

Figure 6: Conceptual links of the characteristics of health governance[160]

– The situation of health financing systems in the African region

---

158 Jacquemot P. Les systèmes de santé en Afrique et l'inégalité face aux soins. *Afrique contemporaine* 2012: 3(243): 95–97.
159 Van Lerberghe W, De Brouwere V. État de santé et santé de l'État en Afrique subsaharienne. *Afrique contemporaine* 2000; 195: 175–190.
160 État de la santé dans la région africaine de l'OMS: analyse de la situation sanitaire, des services et des systèmes de santé dans le contexte des objectifs de développement durable. Organisation mondiale de la Santé, Bureau régional de l'Afrique; 2018.

Health financing systems encompass various methods for mobilising, managing, and using resources. However, 29 countries in the region have not yet developed their health financing strategies. As a result, rather than being proactive, financing in several African countries remains a passive process, with a poorly coordinated structure, form, and outcome[161,162].

*The sources of health financing

Funding for health comes from public, private, or external sources, such as project/programme funds, prepaid funds, or direct payments by users. Public sources are the fairest, external sources are the easiest to target, and private sources are the most sustainable. Public financing covers 7.4 % to 97 % of current health expenditure (as of 2015); external financing covers 0.5 % to 71 %; and private (individual) expenditure covers 2.5 % to 77 % [163,164].

*The management of health funds

Funds for various programmes can be managed in different ways. This can include public programmes, compulsory or voluntary insurance schemes, or direct contributions by individuals. These methods vary considerably from country to country, and each has its own specific management mechanisms[165].

*Service procurement

There are three main approaches for the purchase of health services in the region:

– *Input-based procurement*: This includes recruiting healthcare professionals, constructing infrastructure, and purchasing commodities. All countries in the region use this approach for procuring health services.

---

161 Investir dans la santé en Afrique. Le secteur privé: un partenaire pour améliorer les conditions de vie des populations. Washington: Groupe de la Banque mondiale; 2008.
162 Health system strategy. WHO; 2007. Available at: <http://www.who.int/healthsystems/strategy/en/>
163 État de la santé dans la région africaine de l'OMS: analyse de la situation sanitaire, des services et des systèmes de santé dans le contexte des objectifs de développement durable. Organisation mondiale de la Santé, Bureau régional de l'Afrique; 2018.
164 Investir dans la santé en Afrique. Le secteur privé: un partenaire pour améliorer les conditions de vie des populations. Washington: Groupe de la Banque mondiale; 2008.
165 Health system strategy. WHO; 2007. Available at: <http://www.who.int/healthsystems/strategy/en/>

- *Output-based procurement*: This approach involves funding specific actions such as institutional delivery and childhood vaccination. While it can improve resource utilisation efficiency, it is challenging to develop due to the institutional costs that limit financing.
- *Outcome-based procurement*: Some countries in the region use this approach, particularly in insurance plans or direct payment mechanisms. Financing is based on specific outputs or outcomes, usually defined through diagnostics. The region's experience with this approach is mixed, as it requires significant investment in auditing capacity. It should be noted that each of these approaches has advantages and challenges.
- The situation of information and health research systems in the African region

Information and health research systems consist of all mechanisms for data collection, validation, analysis, and dissemination, as well as knowledge application related to regular health information systems (HIS), vital statistics, research, surveys, and surveillance, and census data sources[166,167,168].

*Health information systems (HIS)

All countries have a HIS for capturing events in healthcare facilities. These systems can be digital (which is a growing trend), paper-based (the most common format) or a combination of both. In many cases, countries have limited to analyse the collected data. Additionally, there is low application of knowledge from HIS, leading decision-makers to generally make decisions without using information from these systems.

*Health surveys and census

Only a small number of countries in the region take proactive measures to plan health surveys, which diminishes the value of this source of health information. Moreover, the content of surveys is typically determined by the financing source rather than by the actual needs on the ground. Furthermore, because these

---

166 État de la santé dans la région africaine de l'OMS: analyse de la situation sanitaire, des services et des systèmes de santé dans le contexte des objectifs de développement durable. Organisation mondiale de la Santé, Bureau régional de l'Afrique; 2018.
167 Health system strategy. WHO; 2007. Available at: <http://www.who.int/healthsystems/strategy/en/>
168 Observatoire mondial de la santé de l'OMS. OMS; 2020.

countries have a limited capacity to analyse survey data, most of the analysis is conducted by external partners.

*Health research

Research is usually initiated by researchers rather than decision-makers, meaning the resulted data generated may not always align with the expectations of those making decisions. Additionally, national research committees often have limited audit capacity, leading to a lack of guidance research processes in many countries. Moreover, research analysis is frequently conducted solely by researchers, with minimal input from the healthcare sector. As a result, translating research findings into policy continues to be a significant challenge in the region.

Chapter 2: African nephrology

1. What is nephrology?

Nephrology is a medical specialty that focusses on preventing, diagnosing, and treating kidney diseases. It is different from urology, which is a surgical speciality dealing with the entire urinary system, including the kidneys, bladder, prostate, and the male genital system.

The term "nephrology" originates from the Greek words "nephrós", meaning kidney, and "lógos", meaning speech or reason.

It should be noted that many diseases affecting the kidneys are not confined to this organ but are general conditions such as high blood pressure, diabetes, and inflammatory diseases.

2. The kidneys: Multifunctional organs

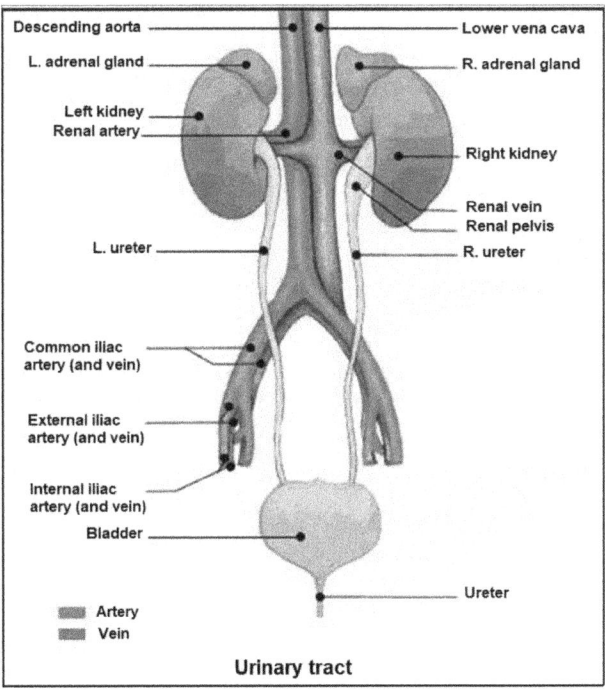

Figure 7: The kidney and the urinary tract

The kidneys are life-sustaining organs that play several vital roles in the body (Figure 7)[169], including:

- Eliminating accumulated toxins;
- Maintaining water, electrolyte and acid-base balance;
- Endocrine (or hormonal) function: producing hormones, enzymes and vitamins such as:

  - Renin, essential for regulating blood pressure;
  - Erythropoietin, involved in red blood cell production;
  - Calcitriol, an active form of vitamin D, crucial for phosphor-calcium and osseous balance.

3. Chronic kidney disease

Chronic kidney disease (CKD) is a significant and fast-growing health issue worldwide.

- A simplified definition of chronic kidney disease:

Chronic kidney disease is defined by the presence, for more than 3 months, of markers of renal damage (such as proteins, blood, or white blood cells at abnormal levels in the urine, along with morphological or renal tissue abnormalities) or a drop in the renal glomerular filtration rate. The renal glomerular filtration rate is the volume of fluid filtered by the kidney per unit time, and helps measure renal activity. The normal flow rate is around 120 ml/min.

Chronic kidney disease is different from acute kidney failure (AKF), which is a rapid onset, potentially reversible decrease in renal filtration rate that can, however, lead to life-threatening, short-term complications. Chronic kidney disease has been classified into 5 stages of increasing severity based on renal glomerular filtration rate and the presence of markers of renal damage. The stage of chronic kidney disease determines the therapeutic management methods[170,171,172].

---

169 Netter FH. *Atlas d'anatomie humaine*. 6e éd. France: Elsevier Masson; 2015.
170 Haddiya I. Focus sur la transplantation rénale. *Revue de médecine générale et de famille* 2010; 10: 86–92.
171 Kidney Disease: Improving Global Outcomes (KDIGO) CKD Work Group. KDIGO 2012 clinical practice guideline for the evaluation and management of chronic kidney disease. *Kidney International* 2013; (suppl 3): 1–150.
172 Recommandations de bonnes pratiques médicales. ALD 17: Insuffisance rénale terminale. SMN; 2013.

– The clinical description and main causes of chronic kidney disease

The severity of chronic kidney disease is closely linked to its silent nature, as clinical signs often do not appear until the disease is in its advanced stages. These signs include toxin accumulation, disturbances in water, electrolyte, and acid-base balance, as well as hormonal function insufficiency. Common signs are asthenia, anorexia, vomiting, nausea, pruritus, anaemia, cardiovascular issues, and phospho-calcium disorders.

The main causes of chronic kidney disease are diabetes mellitus and long-term arterial hypertension. Other causes include primary or secondary glomerular nephropathies, recurring or complicated urinary lithiasis, and hereditary nephropathies like polycystic kidney disease[173].

4. Acute kidney failure

Acute kidney failure (AKF) is the pathological condition that occurs when the kidneys stop working properly, leading to hydro-electrolytic imbalance or an accumulation of body waste. When this happens, it can cause symptoms such as nausea, vomiting, intense fatigue, and anorexia.

There are numerous causes and mechanisms of renal function impairment. Acute kidney failure is a serious medical emergency that can be reversible if managed properly and promptly. Otherwise, it can lead to a permanent damage to the kidneys and eventually result in chronic kidney failure.

5. What is kidney replacement therapy (KRT)?

Kidney replacement therapy involves three main techniques: hemodialysis, peritoneal dialysis, and kidney transplantation.

*When should the replacement therapy be considered?

- In acute kidney failure, replacement therapy depends on the severity of clinical or biological manifestations, such as elevated potassium levels in the blood or metabolic acidosis.
- In chronic kidney disease, initiation of kidney replacement therapy should be considered as soon as the patient reaches stage 5 of the chronic kidney disease, considering the patient's clinical condition, associated comorbidities, and local possibilities.

---

173   Recommandations de bonnes pratiques médicales. ALD 17: Insuffisance rénale terminale. SMN; 2013.

*The informed choice of the replacement therapy

In chronic kidney failure, the patient's choice between different techniques (haemodialysis, peritoneal dialysis, or renal transplantation) should be based on thourough information and explanations. As soon as replacement therapy is considered, the patient should be immediately informed about the potentials, risks, and benefits of kidney transplantation.

Chronic kidney disease, in general, and dialysis, in particular, have a heavy economic impact[174]. For instance, according to the estimates of the Moroccan Society of Nephrology, the annual cost of haemodialysis in Morocco is estimated at 13260 USD per patient . Therefore, the focus should be on preventing kidney disease and developing a culture of kidney transplantation on a larger scale[175].

*Hemodialysis

The human body constantly produces waste products (toxins), which are carried by the blood to the kidneys for purification. In cases of severe renal failure when the kidneys no longer function, an alternative method known as hemodialysis (HD) is used (Figure 8)[176]. This involves filtering the blood outside the body using a machine and an artificial filter called "a dialyser". For patients with chronic renal failure, these sessions last about 4 hours, and are usually done three times a week. To facilitate this process, it is necessary to create a permanent access to the bloodstream in the form of an arteriovenous fistula, which is an ideal vascular access for hemodialysis. The arteriovenous fistula is a connection between an artery and a superficial vein in the forearm or arm, established through surgery. However, it takes several weeks to become fully operational. This technique ensures optimal blood flow for rapid blood filtration, making dialysis possible. In situations where a patient requires urgent hemodialysis but the fistula is not yet in place, dialysis is performed through a central venous catheter. However, the use of this solution can be associated with numerous complications, including the risk of infection.

During the process of hemodialysis, blood is drawn from the body by the machine either through the arteriovenous fistula needle or a central venous

---

174   Eckardt KU et al. Evolving importance of kidney disease: from subspecialty to global health burden. *Lancet* 2013; 382: 158–169.
175   Luyckx VA et al. Equity and economics of kidney disease in sub-Saharan Africa. *Lancet*. 2013; 382: 103–104.
176   La dialyse péritonéale et les autres techniques. RDPLF; 2012. Available at: <https://www.rdplf.org/279-liens-gene-autres-techniques.html>.

catheter. This blood is then pumped through the dialyser to be cleansed, before being injected back into the body through a second needle or a second line of the catheter.

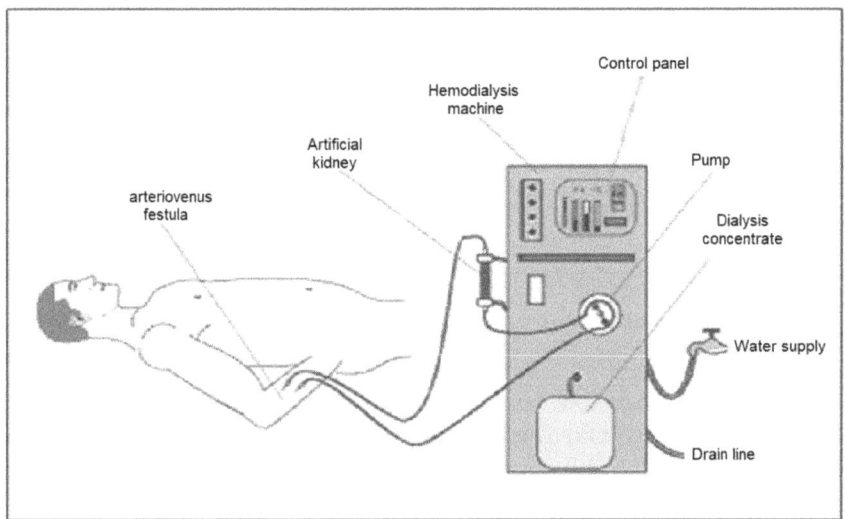

Figure 8: A hemodialysis session- *Peritoneal dialysis and other techniques. RDPLF; 2012.* Available at: <https://www.rdplf.org/279-liens-gene-autres-techniques.html>

*Peritoneal dialysis

Peritoneal dialysis functions on the same principles as hemodialysis. The key difference is that in peritoneal dialysis, the blood is cleansed inside the body by a natural membrane called "the peritoneum", while in hemodialysis, it is cleansed by an artificial membrane (Figure 9)[177]. The peritoneum is a serous membrane of about 2 m², consisting of two layers: one lining inside of the abdominal wall and the other surrounding the organs, with a very significant blood flow at this level. The two layers create a virtual space called "the peritoneal cavity".

---

177   La dialyse péritonéale et les autres techniques. RDPLF; 2012. Available at: <https://www.rdplf.org/279-liens-gene-autres-techniques.html>.

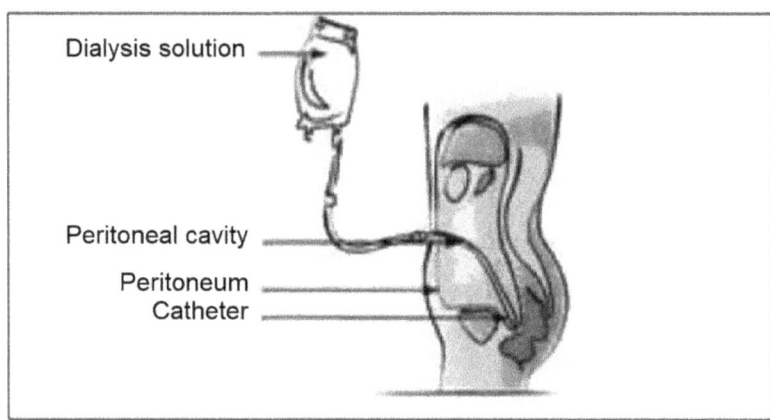

Figure 9: Peritoneal dialysis

Peritoneal dialysis can be done manually or automatically, using the physiological property of the peritoneum's permeability to eliminate excess liquid through ultrafiltration and purify waste through diffusion. To perform dialysis, an artificial liquid called "the dialysate" is introduced into the peritoneal cavity through a surgically implanted catheter in the abdomen. The dialysate removes impurities from the blood plasma as well as excess water, and is then drained after a determined stasis period. This technique offers more patient autonomy compared to hemodialysis and can be performed at home.

*Kidney transplantation

Kidney transplantation is a medical and surgical procedure involving the removal of a kidney from a living or deceased "donor" and its transplantation into a patient with chronic renal failure known as the "recipient". Kidney transplantation is considered the best treatment for chronic renal failure. In most African countries, kidneys for transplant mainly come from related "living donors"[178]. After the transplant, the recipient must take immunosuppressive, anti-rejection drugs daily for the rest of their to prevent organ rejection.

---

178   Ramdani B et al. Consideration on the implementation of a registry of renal transplant recipients and a registry of living donors in the Maghreb countries. *Néphrologie & thérapeutique* 2015; 11(6): 521–524.

– Indications for kidney transplantation

Any patient in stage 5 of chronic end-stage kidney disease, whether on dialysis or not, is a potential candidate for a kidney transplant. Old age is no longer an absolute contraindication.

Generally, transplant candidates undergo dialysis until a suitable kidney becomes available. In some cases, patients may receive a transplant before starting dialysis[179,180,181].

– Contraindications to kidney transplantation

There are no absolute contraindications to kidney transplantation. However, if there are concerns about the patient's adherence to post-transplant therapy, the doctor may advise against the transplant. This is because discontinuing immunosuppressive treatment could result in the rejection of the transplant within a short period of time.

Temporary absolute contraindications include:

– Active infections unless well controlled.
– Invasive cancers.

Additionally, severe cardiovascular, pulmonary, or hepatic diseases pose a high risk of complications or death, making transplantation inadvisable.

6. Nephrology in Africa

Nephrology is often 'overlooked' in the African healthcare system. Costly treatments such as dialysis have been neglected due to the focus on other health priorities such as widespread communicable diseases like tuberculosis and HIV/AIDS, as well as financial mismanagement.

In most African countries, patients with acute kidney disease are rarely treated due to long travel distances, lack of expertise, poverty, and inadequate sustainable funding for health issues. Meanwhile, reports from the African

---

179   Legendre C. *La transplantation rénale*. Paris: Médecine sciences publications Lavoisier; 2012.
180   Matignon M et al. Transplantation rénale: indications, résultats, limites et perspectives. *La Presse médicale* 2007; 36: 1829–1834.
181   Loi n° 16–98 relative au don, au prélèvement et à la transplantation d'organes et de tissus humains . *Bulletin officiel* n: 5480– 15 Kaada 1427 (7-12-2006)

region indicate a constant rise in the number of dialysis patients and those with chronic kidney disease[182].

- African nephrology: The contribution of the African Association of Nephrology (AFRAN) and the International Society of Nephrology (ISN)

In 1987, a group of nephrologists from Egypt, Kenya, Nigeria, Morocco, Tunisia, Algeria, Zambia, Ghana, Tanzania, Uganda, and Sudan established the African Association of Nephrology (AFRAN) to promote and unite African nephrology in terms of training and research. In the same vein, the International Society of Nephrology (ISN) has developed continuing medical education programmes for doctors. It has also created community screening projects in emerging countries, including those in Africa, with significant positive impacts. Consequently, African nephrology has made a notable progress in practice standards since the ISN launched the training fellowship programme three decades ago. In total, the ISN has funded nephrology training for over 100 doctors from several developing African countries, enabling them to work in nephrology units in Europe, Africa, and North America. Most of these beneficiaries were from low- and middle-income countries. Gradually, African doctors are mainly receiving nephrology training in ISN-certified nephrology units based in Africa. This ensures that nephrology graduates gain valuable expertise diagnosing and managing local kidney disease populations using locally available therapy resources.

Over the past decade, 91 % of ISN-sponsored nephrology fellows have returned to their home institutions in Africa, contributing to increased expertise in the management of kidney disease. However, while the ISN fellowship programme has increased the number of nephrologists in Africa, the continent is working on "developing" its own specialists[183,184].

7. Kidney disease in Africa: Epidemiological data

The mismanagement of healthcare funds is prevalent across most parts of Africa. Extreme poverty has further weakened the continent, leading

---

182   Swanepoel CR, Wearne N, Okpechi IG. Nephrology in Africa – not yet uhuru. *Nature Reviews Nephrology* 2013 Oct; 9(10): 610–622.
183   Barsoum RS. History of dialysis in Africa; In Ing TS, Rahman MA, Kjellstrand CM, ed. *Dialysis: history, development and promise.* Singapore: World Scientific Publishing Co.; 2012. pp. 599–610.
184   Barsoum RS, Khalil SS, Arogundade FA. Fifty years of dialysis in Africa: challenges and progress. *American Journal of Kidney Diseases* 2015; 65(3):502–512.

to many death cases among kidney patients due to a lack of access to dialysis[185,186,187].

– Acute kidney failure (AKF) in Africa

It is challenging to interpret data on the incidence of acute kidney failure (AKF) in Africa, given the lack of cohort uniformity, different research outcome compilation methods, and disparities in the diagnosis and treatment of AKF patients across different African countries[188].

Assounga et al.[189] noted that AKF accounted for 0.99 % of all paediatric admissions to a large hospital in Congo-Brazzaville over a five-year period, while Bamgboye et al.[190] from Nigeria found that AKF accounted for 35 % of all admissions in Lagos over a ten-year period. Other researchers found that it represented 4.5 % of all medical admissions in Dakar and 23.2 % of all intensive care units (ICUs) in Cape Town[191]. These rates among patients in hospitals or under emergency care in Africa are higher than those reported in developed countries such as the United States and the United Kingdom, where AKF accounted for 2.5 % of all hospital admissions and 1.34 % of all emergency admissions[192,193].

---

185 Codreanu I, Perico N, Sharma SK et al. Prevention programmes of progressive renal disease in developing nations. *Nephrology* 2006; 11: 321–328.

186 Benghanem Gharbi M et al. Prevalence of chronic kidney disease and associated risk factors: first results from a population based screening program in Morocco (MAREMAR). *Journal of the American Society of Nephrology* 2012; 23: 178A.

187 Abd ElHafeez S, Bolignano D, D'Arrigo G et al. Prevalence and burden of chronic kidney disease among the general population and high-risk groups in Africa: a systematic review. *BMJ Open* 2018; 8: e015069.

188 Swanepoel CR, Wearne N, Okpechi IG. Nephrology in Africa – not yet uhuru. *Nature Reviews Nephrology* 2013 Oct; 9(10): 610–622.

189 Assounga AG, Assambo-Kielim C, Mafoua A, Moyenm G, Nzingoula S. Etiology and outcome of acute renal failure in children in Congo-Brazzaville. *Saudi Journal of Kidney Diseases and Transplantation* 2000; 11: 40–43.

190 Bamgboye EL, Mabayoje MO, Odutola TA, Mabadeje AF. Acute renal failure at the Lagos University Teaching Hospital: a 10-year review. *Renal Failure* 1993; 15: 77–80.

191 Swanepoel CR, Wearne N, Okpechi IG. Nephrology in Africa--not yet uhuru. *Nature Reviews Nephrology* 2013 Oct; 9(10): 610–622.

192 U.S. Renal Data System. USRDS 2012 Annual data report: Atlas of chronic kidney disease and end-stage renal disease in the United States. Bethesda: National Institutes of Health, National Institute of Diabetes and Digestive and Kidney Diseases; 2012.

193 Abraham KA, Thompson EB, Bodger K et al. Inequalities in outcomes of acute kidney injury in England. *QJM*. 2012; 105: 729–740.

It is important to note that the differences in AKF rates between Africa and developed countries may be due to the more accurate data collection and communication in developed countries, as data collection systems in Africa are not well-established and studies lack precision. It may also be due to the variation in patient outcomes depending on the availability of replacement therapy.

- The causes of acute kidney failure (AKF) in Africa

Records showed that severe infection is the primary cause of AKF upon admission to African hospitals. Fewer cases develop AKF after hospitalisation, unlike in developed countries where this often occurs in patients admitted to the hospital with various medical or surgical conditions. Arendse et al.[194] reported that 43.6 % of intensive care unit (ICU) admissions for AKF in HIV-positive patients in Cape Town were due to sepsis. Additionally, Friedericksen et al[195], also from Cape Town, noted that 50 % of ICU AKF cases were due to infections. HIV is a major cause of AKF in Africa due to co-existing infections or the toxicity of medications and their associated complications. Other common, but less reported, causes of AKF in Africa include various nephrotoxic plants, obstetric complications, snake bites, envenomation, and drug abuse leading to malignant hypertension and AKF.

- Challenges in the management of acute kidney failure (AKF)

There are only a few well-equipped ICUs with renal replacement methods for AKF in African urban areas, mostly in North and South Africa. This is due to the lack of specialised infrastructure and funding for this type of therapy in many African countries. Moreover, in many parts of Africa, dialysis is self-funded without government financial assistance. As a result, only a few people can afford treatment, leading to a very high the mortality rate associated with AKF, ranging from 13.3 % to 79.8 % (compared to 12.1 % in the United States)[196,197].

---

194 Arendse C, Okpechi I, Swanepoel C. Acute dialysis in HIV-positive patients in Cape Town, South Africa. *Nephrology* 2011; 16: 39–44.
195 Friedericksen DV, Van der Merwe L, Hattingh TL et al. Acute renal failure in the medical ICU still predictive of high mortality. *South African Medical Journal* 2009; 99: 873–875.
196 Swanepoel CR, Wearne N, Okpechi IG. Nephrology in Africa – not yet uhuru. *Nature Reviews Nephrology* 2013 Oct; 9(10): 610–622.
197 Okunola OO, Ayodele OE, Adekanle AD. Acute kidney injury requiring hemodialysis in the tropics. *Saudi Journal of Kidney Diseases and Transplantation* 2012; 23: 1315–1319.

Peritoneal dialysis (PD), a preferred solution for AKF in Africa due to its lower installation cost compared to hemodialysis, is still hard to introduce in the continent for reasons we will discuss later.

– Chronic kidney disease (CKD) in Africa

Chronic kidney disease is currently one of the major non-communicable diseases worldwide, particularly in low- and middle-income countries. A meta-analysis published in 2014 drew attention to the significance of chronic kidney disease (CKD) in public health in sub-Saharan Africa. This vast territory comprises 85 % (947.4 million) of the total African population[198]. The lowest reported prevalence of CKD (4 %) is in North Africa, particularly in Egypt, Libya, Tunisia, Algeria, and Morocco, while the highest prevalence (16.5 %) is observed in West and Central Africa, which includes Benin, Burkina Faso, Cape Verde, Gambia, Ghana, Guinea, Guinea-Bissau, Côte d'Ivoire, Liberia, Mali, Mauritania, Niger, Nigeria, Cameroon, Senegal, Sierra Leone, São Tomé and Príncipe, and Togo. The average prevalence of CKD for the entire African continent is 10.1 %, while the worldwide prevalence is 13.4 %[199,200]. In Europe, the reported prevalence is lower and more homogeneous: 8.9 % in the Netherlands, 6.8 % in Italy, 5.2 % in Portugal. 4.7 % in Spain and 3.3 % in Norway. The prevalence of CKD in Africa varies widely by region, ranging from 2 % to 41 % in the west/central region, 12 % to 17 % in the central region, 6 % to 29 % in the south, 7 % to 15 % in the east, and 3 % to 13 % in the north. In addition, hypertensive vascular disease is the major cause for CKD in Africa (16 %), followed by diabetic nephropathy (15 %). Africa is the leading continent in infection-induced kidney diseases caused by HIV, hepatitis C, malaria and bilharzia, in addition to nephropathies of toxic or hereditary causes. Finally, it is important to note that the real causes of CKD remain undetermined in one fifth of patients (20 %)[201].

– Treatment options for end-stage kidney disease (ESKD) in Africa

---

198 Codreanu I, Perico N, Sharma SK et al. Prevention programmes of progressive renal disease in developing nations. *Nephrology* 2006; 11: 321–328.
199 Benghanem Gharbi M et al. Prevalence of chronic kidney disease and associated risk factors: first results from a population based screening program in Morocco (MAREMAR). *Journal of the American Society of Nephrology* 2012; 23: 178A.
200 Abd ElHafeez S, Bolignano D, D'Arrigo G, et al. Prevalence and burden of chronic kidney disease among the general population and high-risk groups in Africa: a systematic review. *BMJ Open* 2018; 8: e015069.
201 Swanepoel CR, Wearne N, Okpechi IG. Nephrology in Africa – not yet uhuru. *Nature Reviews Nephrology* 2013 Oct; 9(10): 610–622.

*Hemodialysis

The most widely used replacement therapy in Africa is hemodialysis, which is mainly accessible in big cities. However, the development of this technique has been significantly slowed down in many countries because of poverty, resource mismanagement, and inadequate financing (figure 10).

The average cost of a hemodialysis session in Africa varies considerably, ranging from 30 USD to 100 USD. As more than half of the sub-Saharan population lives on less than 1 USD a day, many patients cannot afford long-term dialysis treatment[202].

In a study involving 158 patients who received treatment for 3 years in Nigeria, Arije et al.[203] showed that 70.9 % of them could only benefit from dialysis for less than a month, compared to only 1.9 % of patients who managed to continue dialysis for more than 12 months. Financial distress resulted in 73.4 % of patients losing their homes after less than 10 hemodialysis sessions. Additional challenges such as the installation of a vascular access (or arteriovenous fistula) for dialysis, access to electricity, water, or transport often become major obstacles for further treatment. Another study revealed that 91.7 % of patients receiving long-term dialysis had only temporary vascular access to dialysis (catheters) due to the lack of vascular surgeons and financial resources, considerably hindering the medium- and long-term hemodialysis treatment[204].

---

202 Barsoum RS, Khalil SS, Arogundade FA. Fifty years of dialysis in Africa: challenges and progress. *American Journal of Kidney Diseases* 2015; 65(3): 502–512.
203 Arije A, Kadiri S, Akinkugbe O. The viability of hemodialysis as a treatment option for renal failure in a developing economy. *African Journal of Medicine and Medical Sciences* 2000; 29: 311–314.
204 Ekpe EE, Ekirikpo U. Challenges of vascular access in a new dialysis centre – Uyo experience. Pan. Afr. Med. 2010; 7: 23.

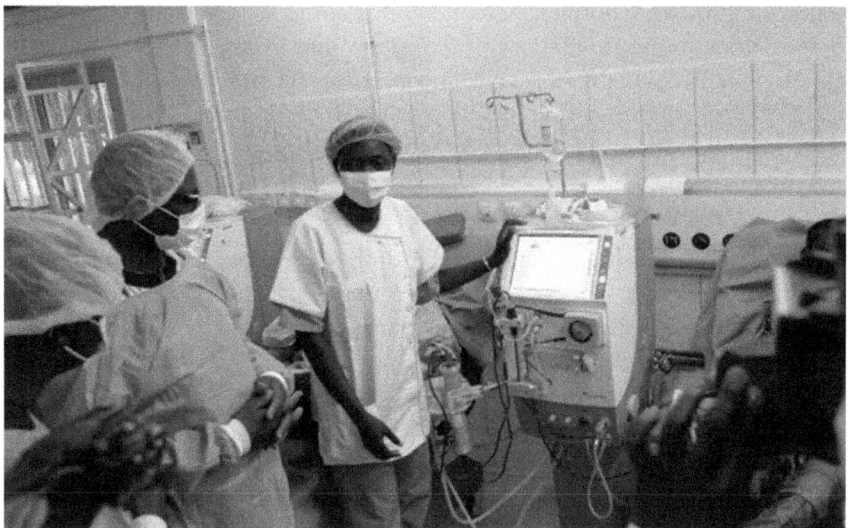

Figure 10: Hemodialysis session in an African Centre (Photo credit: University Hospital Centre – Souro Sanou –Burkina Faso)

*Peritoneal dialysis (PD)

There are a few chronic PD programmes in sub-Saharan African countries. Peritoneal dialysis (PD) can be performed manually without electricity, and is an ideal option for patients in large rural areas in Africa. Unfortunately, importing and transporting PD fluids, as well as dealing with customs formalities, dramatically increase the cost. Even when the fluid is manufactured locally, as is the case in South Africa, it can be as costly as the fluid purchased from foreign suppliers. Additionally, overpopulated environments, lack of adequate water and sanitation, which contributes to increased infections, and low levels of education all make PD impractical in these regions[205].

In the richest countries of North Africa, which service 93 % of the African population on dialysis, PD has been growing very slowly. Only 3 % of all dialysis patients in this region are being treated with this method.

Another barrier to the development of PD is the continued migration of PD-trained staff in search of better opportunities. In addition, due to the shortage of

---

205 Blake PG. PD growth in the developing world. *Peritoneal Dialysis International* 2010; 30: 5–6.

healthcare providers, hospitals are often reluctant to send a health professional for long-term training to master this technique, thus making it harder to provide and promote PD in many African countries. However, despite all the challenges, many PD programmes are successful in Cape Town, Sudan and Senegal, thanks to the help and support of the government.[206].

*Kidney transplantation in Africa

Egypt, Sudan and South Africa are the leading African countries in the number of kidney transplants. Once again, the low numbers of kidney transplants in our continent are due to the high cost of preparing and maintaining this technique and to the lack of infrastructure. The shortage of deceased donors in Africa is accentuated by ethnic and religious beliefs that object to the removal of organs from brain-dead donors. In North Africa, only Morocco, Tunisia, and Algeria perform kidney transplantation from deceased donors.

In many African countries, the costs of transplantation, the laboratory tests required to monitor transplanted patients, and the difficulties in obtaining the necessary medications discourage the practice of kidney transplantation. For instance, due to the high cost of kidney transplantation, which is around 35.000 USD, many patients from Nigeria often travel to India with their donors because the procedure there is less costly[207].

However, many centres in Africa are striving to launch sustainable and innovative programmes. Such is the case of Muller et al. from Groote Schuur Hospital, who started a very successful programme of transplanting HIV-positive patients with kidneys from HIV-positive donors[208].

– The shortage of healthcare providers in Africa

Available data indicate that Africa suffers from a shortage of doctors, especially nephrologists, compared to the rest of the world. "Brain drain" is a serious issue, as skilled and experienced doctors leave Africa to live and work elsewhere. This contributes to the shortage of qualified health professionals across the continent. In some cases, a single nephrologist may be responsible for an entire

---

206 Okpechi I, Rayner BL, Swanepoel C. Peritoneal dialysis in Cape Town, South Africa. *Peritoneal Dialysis International* 2012; 32: 254–260.
207 Swanepoel CR, Wearne N, Okpechi IG. Nephrology in Africa – not yet uhuru. *Nature Reviews Nephrology* 2013 Oct; 9(10): 610–622.
208 Muller E, Barday Z, Mendelson M et al. Renal transplantation between HIV-positive donors and recipients justified. *South African Medical Journal* 2012; 102: 497–498.

population of 2–3 million people. Moreover, in many sub-Saharan countries, administrators without medical qualifications often make health policy and management decisions. The fellowship programme of the International Society of Nephrology (ISN) now requires trainees to return to their home country and work at their home unit for at least three years after completing their training in a host country[209]. Alongside the shortage of healthcare staff, there is also a lack of quality clinical research in nephrology in most African institutions.

In conclusion, Africa a diverse continent with economic, political, and governance differences. It is therefore impossible to use a single approach to address its health situation. Although the health situation is improving along with the continent's economic growth, poverty and mismanagement of healthcare funds make many parts of the continent vulnerable. Kidney disease is a major public health issue, especially in sub-Saharan Africa. Interpreting epidemiological data on this disease is difficult due to the lack of cohort uniformity, absence of registers, and disparities in patient diagnosis and treatment from country to country. The inadequate specialised infrastructure and shortage of qualified healthcare staff, especially nephrologists because of 'brain drain' aggravate the situation of kidney management, resulting in the death of many kidney patients.

In terms of kidney replacement therapy, hemodialysis is the most widely used replacement therapy in Africa, and it is mainly available in big cities. However, inadequate funding has significantly slowed the development of this technique in many African countries. Furthermore, kidney transplantation is still limited in the continent because of the high cost of required laboratory tests, difficulties in obtaining necessary medications, and the lack of suitable infrastructure.

---

209 Harris DCH, Dupuis S, Couser WG et al. Training nephrologists from developing countries: does it have a positive impact? *Kidney International* 2012; Suppl. 2: 275–278.

Part III: Social responsibility in healthcare: An African-wide survey

Chapter 1: An African-wide survey

The primary mission of healthcare facilities is to care for the sick, making social responsibility a crucial aspect in promoting healthcare systems in developed countries. Many studies in the United States, Europe, and Asia focus on the concept of "socially responsible" healthcare, which refers to a system that provides quality care in alignment with the needs of the population. In this regard, it is essential to examine the healthcare situation in Africa: Are the African healthcare systems socially responsible in managing kidney disease, which can be particularly costly? How do African healthcare professionals, especially nephrologists, perceive hospitals and the healthcare systems more globally? Are African kidney patients satisfied with the existing healthcare facilities, and do they consider them "socially responsible"? Furthermore, what factors influence the perceptions of patients and caregivers regarding social responsibility in renal healthcare across the continent? And, finally, what practical suggestions can be made to enhance the social responsibility of African healthcare systems, especially in the management of kidney disease?

The absence of African research on this subject led us to examine social responsibility regarding the situation of renal healthcare in Africa from the perspectives of patients and nephrologists. Conducting this survey-based analysis can help us pinpoint the factors influencing these perceptions and formulate proposals for improvement.

Our survey took place over a one-year period between February 2019 and February 2020, and included African patients and nephrologists working in public regional and/or university hospitals with clinical nephrology, dialysis and/or renal transplantation services in Africa.

We narrowed down our research to the social responsibility of hospitals from a "professional responsibility" perspective, based on suggestions from experts and findings from previous studies[210,211]. Specifically, we examined the obligation of hospitals to effectively fulfil their health care role, meet legal, ethical, and philanthropic expectations, and adhere to the principles of quality, equity,

---

210 La Rosa E, Dubois G, Tonnellier F. Social responsibility in health and the global health situation: towards new health and social indicators. *Revue de santé publique* 2007; 19(3): 217–27.

211 Liu W, Shi L, Pong RW et al. How patients think about social responsibility of public hospitals in China?. *BMC Health Services Research* 2016; 16: 371.

pertinence, and efficiency in their care delivery. To measure the perceptions of patients and nephrologists regarding the hospital's performance, we developed two structured questionnaires based on four dimensions:

(i) The quality of service: This includes the therapeutic management and treatment effects, hospital environment, and the care process, such as how patients are kept updated about their illness and treatment, therapeutic protocols, and attentiveness of their caregivers.
(ii) The pertinence of care: This covers the patient's medical history, clinical examination, and medical prescriptions.
(iii) Accessibility: This refers to the availability of health services, including accessibility to treatment, reasonable waiting times for consultations or hospitalisation, and affordable costs of treatment and different tests.
(iv) Professional ethics: This involves providing equitable care and access to treatment regardless of patients' ability to pay. It also involves ensuring patients' privacy and data protection.

The items above were evaluated using a 5-point Likert scale, and the participating doctors answered open-ended questions. We used these questions to better understand their perceptions of hospitals' social responsibility in managing kidney disease. The questions targeted the quality of care, equity in care delivery, and healthcare ethics, which encompasses the principles of justice and beneficence. We also asked the doctors about the barriers to social responsibility in their institutions and invited them to suggest practical solutions.

We assessed the internal validity of our questionnaires avoid any internal consistency bias that might affect the results. We also used Cronbach's alpha index to measure the internal consistency or reliability of the Lickert scale. This index ranged between 0.8 and 0.87 among patients and doctors, indicating good internal consistency of the questionnaire.

For statistical analysis, we used Student t-test, Chi-square test, as well as univariate and multivariate logistic regression methods on several levels. The objective was to examine the factors influencing the patients' and nephrologists' evaluation of hospital social responsibility. A value of $p<0.05$ was considered significant.

Chapter 2: Patients: The characteristics and perceptions of hospital social responsibility

1. The selected patients: Recruitment challenges

Our initial goal was to include a total number of 500 patients with the consent of the lead nephrologists affiliated with each selected centre in the following countries:

- North Africa: Morocco, Egypt, Tunisia
- West Africa: Mauritania, Mali, Senegal
- East Africa: Ethiopia, Kenya, Rwanda, Burundi
- Central Africa: Cameroon, Gabon, Chad
- Southern Africa: South Africa, Zambia, Mozambique

However, during data collection, some principal investigators were unable to provide patient data due to challenges in translating the questionnaire into local dialect and a the lack of research assistants to help illiterate patients. Additionally, some investigators faced obstacles due to regulations imposed by their institutions' ethics committees.

Despite all these challenges, our study successfully included 310 patients from the following African countries (figures 11):

- North Africa (43.87 %): Morocco 32.6 %, Tunisia 5.2 %, Egypt 6.1 %.
- Central Africa (25.81 %): Chad 10.3 %, Cameroon 5.8 %, Gabon 9.7
- West Africa (16.13 %): Mauritania 11.3 %, Senegal 4.8
- Southern Africa (5.48 %): Mozambique: 5.5 %.
- East Africa (8.71 %): Burundi 8.7 %,

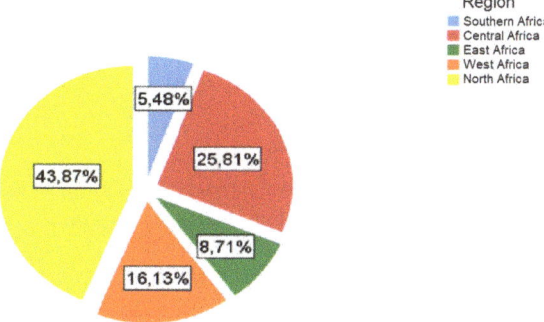

Figure 11: A diagram illustrating the regions of patient affiliation

Despite the strong support from many African nephrologists for our study, we encountered similar difficulties as reported in previous works investigating research obstacles in Africa. The African environment is often considered "not conducive" to research due to various challenges such as[212,213]:

- The lack of motivated, skilled, and determined health workforce. The few doctors and health professionals working in African hospitals are overwhelmed by clinical tasks and workload. Sub-Saharan Africa has less than 1 % of the world's financial resources for the health sector and only 3 % of the world's health workforce. Health researchers are poorly paid and often demotivated by the lack of career opportunities. In addition, the lack of proper leadership of research teams and the issue of brain drain are serious barriers to be considered.
- The financial barriers and logistical challenges, such as limited or unreliable internet access, were frequently reported.
- Regulations at the national or hospital level , including challenges with securing the approval of ethics committees should also be highlighted. Some of these committees asked for payment for their services, which was often a deterrent for unfunded research.

It is essential to have competent and operational research ethics committees, as well as the support of governments and of other donors to establish and promote research in the continent[214].

In response to the constraints mentioned above, we decided to reduce the total number of questions in the various questionnaires, which would take between 10 and 15 minutes of the patient's time. The investigators were unable to use longer questionnaires due to staff shortage, as it would have been too burdensome.

---

212 Conradie A, Duys R, Forget P et al. Barriers to clinical research in Africa: a quantitative and qualitative survey of clinical researchers in 27 African countries. *British Journal of Anaesthesia* 2018; 121(4): 813e821.
213 Whitworth JA, Kokwaro G, Kinyanjui S et al. Strengthening capacity for health research in Africa. *Lancet* 2008; 372: 1590e3.
214 Van Hoving DJ, Brysiewicz P. African emergency care providers' attitudes and practices towards research. *African Journal of Emergency Medicine* 2017; 7: 9e14.

2. The socio-economic characteristics of the selected countries

Table 2 displays the socioeconomic characteristics of the ten countries included in our study, based on the World Bank's indicators[215].

Table 2: The socio-economic characteristics of the targeted countries

Country	Surface area (km²)	Population (in millions)	GDP: (in billion USD)	GNP: (in dollars PPP)	Healthcare expenditure per capita (PRPP USD)	Public expenditure on education (in %GDP)	Public expenditure healthcare (in %GDP)	Population with access to improved drinking water (%)	Population with access to adequate sanitation (%)
Chad	1284000	14.9	9,981	1920	79,00	28,96	3,60	43,00	10,00
Egypt	997739	97.55	235,400	11360	594,00	3,80	5,60	99,30	94,70
Cameroon	475650	23.799	38,502	3640	122,00	3,60	4,10	61,00	40,40
Senegal	196839	15.85	16,370	2620	107,00	6,20	4,70	78,60	70,00
Gabon	267668	20.25	14,620	17010	599,00	2,67	3,40	66,00	41,90
Tunisia	163610	11.53	40,260	132	785,00	6,60	7,10	93,00	85,00
Morocco	710850	35.74	109,100	8063	447,00	5,26	5,90	83,00	86,00
Mozambique	801590	29.67	12,330	1200	79,00	6,50	7,00	57,00	20,00
Burundi	27834	10.86	3,478	770	58,00	4,34	7,50	71,00	68,00
Mauritania	1030000	4.42	5,025	3900.00	148.00	2.60	3.80	68.00	40.00

GDP: Gross domestic product; GNP: Gross national product; PPP: Purchasing power parity; PRPP: Production power parity USD: US dollar.

– The classification of the selected countries by income

We selected ten countries from the five regions in Africa, categorised into three groups by the World Bank (Table 3)[216]:

– Upper-middle income countries
– Lower middle-income countries
– Low-income countries

---

215 La banque mondiale: Indicateurs 2020. Banque mondiale; 2020. Available at: <https://donnees.banquemondiale.org/indicateur>.
216 La banque mondiale: Indicateurs 2020. Banque mondiale; 2020. Available at: <https://donnees.banquemondiale.org/indicateur>.

Table 3: A breakdown of the targeted countries according to the World Bank classification

Country	Classification by income level
Maroc	Lower middle-income countries
Tunisie	
Égypte	
Sénégal	
Mauritanie	
Cameroun	
Gabon	Upper-middle income countries
Tchad	Low-income countries
Burundi	
Mozambique	

- The classification of the selected countries in terms of healthcare and education expenditure:

Table 4 shows the classification of the selected countries based on their healthcare expenditure and education expenditure per capita.

Table 4: Classification of the targeted countries according to their healthcare and education expenditure

Healthcare expenditure per capita (PRPP USD)	Countries
<100	Burundi- Mozambique- Chad
100–300	Cameroon-Senegal-Mauritania
300–500	Morocco
500–700	Egypt-Gabon
700–800	Tunisia
Public expenditure on education (in % GDP)	
<5 %	Egypt-Cameroon-Gabon-Burundi-Mauritania
5–10 %	Morocco- Mozambique- Tunisia- Senegal
>10 %	Chad

PRPP: Production power parity; USD: US dollar; GDP: Gross domestic product

3. The provision of nephrology care by country

Table 5 shows the availability of nephrology care in the surveyed countries. In North Africa, the density of nephrologists exceeds 10 per million population, while in the other African regions, density is less than 5 per million population. Hemodialysis is available in all the selected countries, but peritoneal dialysis is only offered in five ones (Morocco, Tunisia, Egypt, Senegal and Mozambique). As for kidney transplantation, it is only performed in three North African countries (Morocco, Tunisia, and Egypt).

Table 5: The provision of nephrology care by country

Country	Density of nephrologists (PMP)	Number of nephrology centres	Prevalence of treated ESKD (PMP)	Number of chronic hemodialysis patients (CHD)	PD activity	KT activity
Morocco	10.1– 15	Public 110 Private 236 Associative 38	433–759	32000	Yes	Yes
Tunisia	>15	Public 12	759.1 – 1048	N/A	Yes	Yes
Egypt	>15	Total 500 Public N/A Private N/A	433–759	70000	Yes	Yes
Mauritania	10	Public 13 Private 2	N/A	1030	No	No
Senegal	<5	Public 22 Private 4	N/A	N/A	Yes	No
Cameroon	<5	Public 8 Private 3	N/A	1300	No	No
Gabon	ND	Public 2 Private 5	N/A	N/A	Non	No
Chad	0.26	Public 2	N/A	90	No	No
Burundi	0.19	Public 2	N/A	60	No	No
Mozambique	0.08	N/A	N/A	N/A	Yes	No

N/A: Not available; ECKF: end-stage chronic kidney failure; CHD: Chronic hemodialysis patient; KD: Kidney transplantation; PMP: Per million population.

4. Patient demographics

Age: In our study, most patients were young, with a mean age of 46.51 ± 14.67, and ages ranging from 17 to 84. Also, 90.73 % of the participants were under 65 years of age, and the most represented age group was adults between 45 and 55 (21.9 %). In Southern Africa, the most represented age group was those between 35 and 45, constituting 52.9 % of all participants from this region. In Cameroon, Gabon, and Mauritania, the youngest age group was 25–35, making up 33.3 %, 30 %, and 25.7 % respectively.

These results differ significantly from literature data, particularly, from Western sources which confirm that the prevalence of chronic kidney disease increases considerably with age[217]. High prevalence of chronic kidney disease among the elderly indicates a range of risk factors such as diabetes and hypertension, in addition to an age-related decline of renal function[218]. According to a key American survey (NHANES), over a third of people over 70 had moderate or severe chronic kidney disease[219]. A large French multicentre study found that the mean age of French dialysis patients was 65.9 +/-14.5[220]. Another American multicentre study including 10,137 chronic hemodialysis patients reported a median age of 63, with 48.8 % of patients over 68 of age[221].

In our study, the patients were generally younger compared to those studied in wealthier countries. Previous research has indicated that in Africa, especially in sub-Saharan Africa, chronic kidney disease tends to impact individuals aged 20–50, who are potentially active and economically productive[222]. This can be attributed to African demographics, as the age distribution in Africa is characterised by a broad base and a narrow top, resulting in a low percentage of individuals over 60. It is worth noting that Africa has the youngest population in the world. Furthermore, the continent's young population is growing rapidly, as it is projected that by 2055, people aged 15–24 will be more than double the 2015 total of 226 million. Still, in North Africa, the young population is starting to decline[223,224,225]

The incidence of kidney disease among young people in Africa can also be attributed to HIV-associated kidney damage, tuberculosis, and malaria which, in

---

217   Prakash S, O'Hare AM. Interaction of Aging and CKD. Semin Nephrol. 2009; 29(5): 497–503.
218   Population Finder. United States Census Bureau; 2008. Available at: from:<http://factfinder.census.gov/servlet/SAFFPopulation?_sse=on
219   Coresh J et al. Prevalence of chronic kidney disease in the United States. *JAMA* 2007; 298(17): 2038–2047.
220   Nguyen Thi PL, Frimat L, Loos-Ayav C. SDIALOR: A dialysis patient satisfaction questionnaire. *Néphrologie & Thérapeutique* 2008; 4: 266–277.
221   Richardson MM, Paine SS, Grobert ME, Satisfaction with care of patients on hemodialysis. *Clinical Journal of the American Society of Nephrology* 2015; 10(8): 1428–1434.
222   Lacson E Jr., Wang W, Lazarus JM et al. Hemodialysis facility-based quality-of-care indicators and facility-specific patient outcomes. *American Journal of Kidney Diseases* 2009; 54: 490–497.
223   Yahia M. Africa's defining challenge. Africa: UNDP; 2017.
224   Rural Development Report Creating opportunities for rural youth. Rome: IFAD (International Fund for Agricultural Development); 2019.
225   Revision of World Population Prospects. World Economic Forum. United Nations; 2019.

addition to diabetes and hypertension, pose significant challenges to healthcare systems in sub-Saharan Africa. Additionally, specialised management of kidney disease to slow its progression towards chronicity and terminal stage is not always available in many African countries, further adding to the burden of kidney disease[226].

***Gender**: The majority of the participating patients were male (58.77 % male and 41.23 % female), resulting in a M/F sex ratio of 1.42. In Southern Africa, there was a high percentage of female patients (64.7 % vs. 35.3 %), whereas other African regions showed a male predominance. Female predominance was also observed in Cameroon (66.7 %), Mauritania (60 %), Mozambique (64.7 %), and Tunisia (53.3 %).

Gender plays a well-known factor in determining the risk of developing, progressing, and experiencing complications from chronic kidney disease. Women tend to have a higher risk of developing the disease, when mean tend to experience more severe forms[227]. In Europe, the M/F sex ratio is 0.96[228]. A study conducted in France on dialysis patient satisfaction revealed that 60.3 % of the participants were men. The study authors noted that women seemed to be less responsive to questionnaires, a trend observed in other studies as well[229]. This observation raises the possibility of a selection bias, which should be considered when interpreting the study results.

Other large-scale studies in Europe and the Americas , focussing on a substantial number of patients with renal failure or undergoing chronic hemodialysis, also found a male predominance in 55 % and 55.5 % of cases, respectively[230,231]. These rates align with those in our study. Still, it is important

---

226 Van Biesen W, Jha V, Abu-Alfa AK. Considerations on equity in management of end-stage kidney disease in low- and middle-income countries. *Kidney International Supplements* 2020; 10: e63–e71.
227 Abd ElHafeez S, Bolignano D, D'Arrigo G, et al. Prevalence and burden of chronic kidney disease among the general population and high-risk groups in Africa: a systematic review. *BMJ Open* 2018; 8: e015069.
228 European Union Sex ratio. Index mundi, CIA World Factbook; 2018. Available at: <https://www.indexmundi.com/european_union/sex_ratio.html>
229 Nguyen Thi PL, Frimat L, Loos-Ayav C. SDIALOR: A dialysis patient satisfaction questionnaire. *Néphrologie & Thérapeutique* 2008; 4: 266–277.
230 Palmer SC, de Berardis G, Craig JC et al. Patient satisfaction with in-centre haemodialysis care: an international survey. *BMJ Open* 2014; 4: e005020.
231 Richardson MM, Paine SS, Grobert ME, Satisfaction with care of patients on hemodialysis. *Clinical Journal of the American Society of Nephrology* 2015; 10(8): 1428–1434.

to interpret them within the African context where the M/F sex ratio at birth generally varies between 1 and 1.06, depending on country and region[232]:

- North Africa: 1.05 – 1.06
- Southern Africa: 1 – 1.03
- West Africa: 1.03 – 1.05
- East Africa: 1.02 – 1.03
- Central Africa: 1.02 – 1.03

The sex ratio in different countries is influenced by a variety of factors such as the country's history, social structure, and economic conditions. For example, during the first two years following the 1994 genocide in Rwanda, women made up 70 % of the adult population due to the loss of a large number of men. Similarly, women outnumber men in countries like Namibia, Mozambique, and Senegal possibly due to male migrations to foreign countries[233].

It is important to note that women in Africa do not always have access to healthcare, which can also explain male predominance in our survey. A report by the WHO revealed that in many African countries, the poorest individuals, especially women, are the most impacted by inadequate healthcare systems and bear the cost of health services. Women often rely on men for financial support to access healthcare, leading to inadequate care, especially for expensive treatments like kidney disease.

5. Patients' socio-economic data

After considering the non-modifiable factors of age and gender that influence health, we will now focus on the socio-economic factors affecting our patients, which are known as the social determinants of health. These factors account for inequalities in healthcare status and access among people of different social levels[234,235]. It is widely acknowledged that economic and social conditions

---

232 Sex Ratio in Africa. African development Bank Group; Aug. 2019. Available at: <https://dataportal.opendataforafrica.org/ouhoojg/sex-ratio-in-africa>
233 Mungai C. Sex ratios in Africa: where women outnumber men, and vice versa, and why it matters. Africa pedia; 2017. Available at: <https://africapedia.com/sex-ratio-africa/>
234 Walker RJ, Smalls BL, Campbell JA et al. Impact of social determinants of health on outcomes for type 2 diabetes: a systematic review. *Endocrine*. 2014 Sept; 47(1): 29–48.
235 Blane D et al. Disease etiology and materialist explanations of socioeconomic mortality differentials. *European Journal of Public Health* 1997; 7: 385–391.

significantly impact individuals' lifelong health. The poor are at least twice as likely to suffer from serious illness or premature death than the rich. The overall health status of the population varies continuously between these two extremes, . Therefore, health policies should be developed in consideration of these determinants[236].

– Place of residence

The world is rapidly is quickly becoming more urbanised with a growing population since the late 2000s. However, Africa, especially sub-Saharan Africa, still has a significant rural population. In 2015, about 62 % of Africans were living in rural areas. This is because urbanisation in the region is a relatively recent phenomenon, and it may not reach the urban-rural tipping point until the late 2030s[237]. Burundi has the highest rural population, with 86.97 % of the total population, while Gabon has the lowest rate, with only 10.63 % of the total population[238].

It was found out that 74.7 % of the targeted patients were living in urban areas, while 25.3 % were living in rural areas. This pattern was consistent across all African regions and countries included in the study. This raises concerns about the access to specialised nephrology care for rural populations. Generally, access to healthcare services is generally more challenging for rural communities worldwide, as health facilities are usually concentrated in cities and regional centres. Consequently, rural and remote populations tend to have lower life expectancy and poorer health status compared to their urban counterparts. Furthermore, there is a global shortage of health professionals, which is more prominent in rural areas of poor and developing countries. This is particularly true for a vast continent like Africa, which has a relatively underdeveloped health infrastructure[239]. For example, the healthcare system in Ghana only serves

---

236   Wunch G et al. Socioeconomic differences in mortality: a life course approach. *European Journal of Population* 1996; 12: 167–185.
237   Mercandalli S, Losch B. *Rural Africa in motion. Dynamics and drivers of migration South of the Sahara*. Rome: FAO and CIRAD; 2017.
238   World Bank staff estimates based on the United Nations Population Division's World Urbanization Prospects. World Bank; 2018.
      Available at:<https://www.indexmundi.com/facts/indicators/SP.RUR.TOTL.ZS/map/africa>.
239   Strasser R, Kam SM, Regalado SM. Rural health care access and policy in developing countries. *Annual Review of Public Health* 2016; 37: 395–412.

less than 50 % of the rural population, highlighting the inequity in access to healthcare based on place of residence[240].

– Income

Poverty is considered a significant factor affecting access to healthcare. It is not only about lack of income or material possessions, but also about the inability to live a fulfilling life. Despite improvements in global healthcare access in the past decade, there are still significant gaps, especially for the poorest people[241].

Africa is the continent with the highest levels of poverty. Currently, one in three Africans (or 422 million people) live below the global poverty line, constituting more than 70 % of the world's poorest people. Nevertheless, according to projections from the World Data Lab, Africa has now reached an important milestone in the fight against poverty[242].

Additionally, over the past two decades, the economic landscape in Africa has undergone significant change, marked by an average annual growth of 5.5 % from 2001 to 2015. The traditional divide of a small wealthy minority and a large poor majority no longer characterises the African population. A burgeoning has emerged representing nearly one-third of the total African population . It consists of individuals with a daily income between 2 USD and 20 USD,[243,244]. However, this income-based definition has its limitations as it does not fully capture the diverse dynamics and socio-economic realities of each country.

It was also found that 46.26 % of the surveyed patients reported having a low income, with a majority located in Cameroon (62.5 %), Morocco (58.7 %), Mauritania (52.9 %), and Tunisia (62.5 %). Next, 43.54 % reported having a medium income, primarily from Burundi (63 %), Egypt (42.1 %), Gabon (63.3 %),

---

240 Lavy V, Strauss J, Duncan Thomas et al. Quality of health care, survival and health outcomes in Ghana. *Journal of Health Economics* 1996; 15: 333–357.
241 Ortiz-Prado E, Ponce J, Cornejo-Leon F et al. Analysis of health and drug access associated with the purchasing power of the Ecuadorian population. *Global Journal of Health Science* 2017; 9(1): 201–210.
242 Hamel K, Tong, Hofer M. Poverty in Africa is now falling – but not fast enough. Brookings 2019.
243 AFDB, "The Middle of the Pyramid, Dynamics of the Middle class in Africa", Mar. 2011.
244 The middle class in Africa realities and challenges. CFAO; 2015. Available at: <http://www.cfaogroup.com/static/2017/12/08/CFAO-White%20Paper%20The%20middle%20classes%20in%20Africa%20UK%20april2016.pdf?qA3g3_m5sGX6zBNHJgp4PQ:qA3g3_m5sGX6zBNHJgp4PQ:flcrNtDaj1kHsdVnXP2w9g>.

Senegal (46.7 %), and Chad (50 %). Only 10.20 % of patients reported having a high income.

Income is one of the key social determinants of health that significantly impacts access to healthcare. A report from Africa indicated that in Nigeria, the minimum yearly income needed to sustain a basic standard of living is 1,016 USD per year in urban areas and 758 USD in rural areas. However, 74 % of Nigerians live below this income threshold, with 40 % living below the poverty line[245].

Our survey revealed varying income levels among patients in different countries. For instance, in Cameroon, Morocco, Mauritania, and Tunisia, many low-income patients have access to renal care in public hospitals. By contrast, in Burundi, Chad, Egypt, Gabon, Senegal, and Mozambique, most patients receiving this expensive care in public hospitals have average or high incomes. This raises important questions about access to healthcare for low-income patients in these countries and whether they can afford the associated costs.

The report from Nigeria offers insights into our questions regarding healthcare costs. It estimates that the average cost for the initial treatment of chronic kidney failure (CKF) at the start of a dialysis programme is 431 USD. This burdensome cost makes access to this treatment or long-term adherence almost impossible[246].

Access to healthcare in these extremely limited-resource settings therefore greatly depends on the availability of health coverage and the universality of this coverage in the targeted countries, as will be discussed below. This highlights the fact that access to healthcare for poor African populations remains limited and continues to be an unresolved issue[247].

– The availability of health coverage

According to a WHO report, half of the world's population lacks access to full social protection. Access to healthcare is a main concern for people in poor and developing countries. Every year 100 million people are pushed into poverty and 150 million people suffer from impoverishment or financial catastrophe due to out-of-pocket expenditure on health services and the lack of universal health coverage[248].

---

245 Report: Income Inequality Skewed Wealth, Resources to Pockets of 20 % of Nigerians. This Day Business Newspaper June 2016.
246 Blane D et al. Disease etiology and materialist explanations of socioeconomic mortality differentials. *European Journal of Public Health* 1997; 7: 385–391 .
247 Soors et al. Lack of access to health care for African indigents: a social exclusion perspective. *International Journal for Equity in Health* 2013; 12: 91.
248 Universal Health coverage. Regional office for Africa,WHO; 2019.

In developed countries, an estimated 23 million adults in the United States do not have health insurance, while in other countries such as Canada, the Netherlands, and the United Kingdom, healthcare systems do not require cost-sharing for primary care. In France, low-income adults and those with chronic diseases are exempt from out-of-pocket spending, and in Germany such spending is capped at 1 % of income for the chronically ill[249].

In Africa, 60–70 % of the health expenses are paid by households, compared to a global average of 46 %. Many African people still have unmet health needs because health insurance only covers a small percentage of patients[250,251], leading to gaps and inequalities in access to healthcare both within and between countries[252,253]. As for kidney disease, over 80 % of patients receiving treatment for kidney failure live in wealthy countries with universal healthcare access. In contrast, the majority of patients in developing countries cannot afford this treatment. African countries bear a heavy burden because the social security or health insurance systems cannot meet the enormous financial demands placed on patients and their families[254].

In our study, 64.77 % of patients received health coverage, which was publicly funded in 83.44 % of the cases. It is important to note that public health insurance varies in terms of the medical benefits it provides. For example, in Morocco, the Medical Assistance Regime for the Economically Unprivileged (RAMED), based on the principles of social assistance and national solidarity for the poor, covers the costs of treatment in public hospitals and health services. However, it does not include treatments such as the anti-rejection drugs needed by kidney transplant patients.

---

249   Osborn R, Squires D, Doty MM et al. In New survey of eleven countries, US adults still struggle with access to and affordability of health care. *Health Affairs* 2016; 35(12): 2327–2336.
250   Adejumo OA, Akinbodewa AA, Ogunleye A et al. Cost implication of inpatient care of chronic kidney disease patients in a tertiary hospital in Southwest Nigeria. *Saudi Journal of Kidney Diseases and Transplantation* 2020; 31: 209–214.
251   Riman HB, Akpan ES. Healthcare financing and health outcomes in Nigeria: A state level study using multivariate analysis. *International Journal of Humanities and Social Science* 2012; 15: 296–309.
252   Report: Income Inequality Skewed Wealth, Resources to Pockets of 20 % of Nigerians. This Day Business Newspaper June 2016.
253   Riman HB, Akpan ES. Healthcare financing and health outcomes in Nigeria: a state level study using multivariate analysis. *International Journal of Humanities and Social Science* 2012; 15: 296–309.
254   Dechambenoit G. Access to health care in sub-Saharan Africa. *Surgical Neurology International* 2016; 7: 108.

Additionally, at the regional level, 64.7 % of patients in Southern Africa, 55.1 % in Central Africa, and 69.6 % in West Africa had no health coverage. At the country level, 88.9 % of the enrolled patients from Cameroon, 64.5 % from Mauritania, 64.7 % from Mozambique, 80 % from Senegal, and 90 % from Chad had no health coverage.

Based on this data, it can be inferred that the patients in our study faced difficulties in accessing healthcare, particularly renal care, due to the lack of health coverage. This could explain why, despite the low proportion of patients with health coverage across the African continent, 64.77 % of the participants in our survey had some form of health coverage.

Ensuring equitable access to healthcare requires the establishment of **Universal Health Coverage** (UHC). This means that everyone should be able to obtain high-quality healthcare services, including health promotion, preventive, curative, palliative, and rehabilitative without experiencing financial hardship. The attainment of Universal health coverage is also one of the Sustainable Development Goals adopted by the United Nations General Assembly in 2015. However, the successful implementation of UHC requires robust healthcare systems and substantial funding[255]. In wealthier countries, the average per capita health expenditure is estimated at 3,100 USD, while, in sub-Saharan Africa, it is 37 USD. Additionally, the healthcare budget of a country with a population of 10 million is equivalent to the budget of a regional health centre serving 100.000 people in a developed country[256].

It should be noted that African countries face significant social and economic challenges in areas like infrastructure, health, education, and security. These challenges are compounded by limited financial resources. However, several African countries, including Senegal, Ghana, Gabon, the Ivory Coast, Kenya, and Benin have begun to overcome these hurdles by introducing various types of universal health insurance coverage.

– The educational level

A study conducted in Ghana[257] noted that families with an educated head or spouse were healthier than those with illiterate parents. This finding is interesting given that sub-Saharan Africa has the highest rate of school exclusion in the world.

---

255 Universal Health coverage. Regional office for Africa. WHO; 2019.
256 Dechambenoit G. Access to health care in sub-Saharan Africa. *Surgical Neurology International* 2016; 7: 108.
257 Lavy V, Strauss J, Duncan Thomas et al. Quality of health care, survival and health outcomes in Ghana. *Journal of Health Economics* 1996; 15: 333–357.

More than a fifth of 6–11 years-olds, a third of 12–14-year-olds, and about 60 % of 15–17-year-olds remain out of school[258]. According to UNESCO[259], there have been some increases in primary school enrolment in the continent over the last few decades, but inequalities and dysfunctions still persist. Similar to healthcare, access to education also disproportionately impacts the most vulnerable groups[260].

A multicentre study involving European and American hemodialysis patients found that 40.2 % of patients had an educational level of 6–8 years[261].

In our study, 23.21 % of the patients included had no schooling, 21.16 % attended primary school, 31.40 % attended secondary school, and 24.23 % had been to a university.

The majority of patients with a university level (86.7 %) belonged to the region of Southern Africa; those from Central and North Africa had a secondary level (40.5 % and 33.1 % respectively); patients from East Africa had a primary level (63 %), and patients from West Africa were illiterate (37.5 %).

These findings might indicate that access to healthcare is more difficult for the less educated people in sub-Saharan Africa. This is supported by studies of kidney patients in the region, which have noted that participants with higher levels of education, particularly the university level, are more acknowledgeable about common health problems and more likely seek hospital care, understand and adhere to physicians' therapeutic instructions. Moreover, the former might have better economic conditions and thus more likely to seek and comply with hospital care[262].

6. Patients' renal data

– Patient types

In our study, 29.93 % of patients were inpatients while 70.07 % were outpatients (seen in consultation or receiving chronic hemodialysis sessions). The majority

---

258 Sud N. Health and education in Africa. World Bank group; 2020. Available at: <https://www.ifc.org/wps/wcm/connect/REGION__EXT_Content/Regions/Sub-Saharan+Africa/Investments/HealthEducation/>.
259 Education in Africa. UNESCO Institute of Statistics; 2020.
260 Musau Z. Africa grapples with huge disparities in education. Africa renewal; 2018.
261 Palmer SC, de Berardis G, Craig JC et al. Patient satisfaction with in-centre haemodialysis care: an international survey. *BMJ Open* 2014; 4: e005020.
262 Halle MP, Nyongbella J, Fouda H et al. Factors associated with late presentation of patients with chronic kidney disease in nephrology consultation in Cameroon-a descriptive cross-sectional study. *Renal Failure* 2019; 41(1): 384–392.

of the participating patients in all African countries were either outpatients or receiving hemodialysis. In Mauritania and Chad, the majority were inpatients, accounting for 51.5 % vs. 48.5 % and 63.6 % vs. 36.4 % respectively. Additionally, 83.6 % of included patients had chronic renal failure, while 16.4 % were hospitalised for acute kidney failure.

The studies similar to ours, conducted in China, found that there were more outpatients than inpatients, although no explanation was given for this finding. A similar trend was noted in a survey of the care satisfaction of 10,137 American renal failure patients, which revealed that 72.7 % of them were not hospitalised. It was observed that those who agreed to participate in the survey were generally in stable and relatively good health, and were not hospitalised. Additionally, the nursing staff tended to focus on patients who were relatively well and hesitated to include impaired patients in the studies. However, these differences in patient types were not found to influence the questionnaire responses.

In the context of kidney disease, patients in need of hospitalisation often experience asthenia and a worsening of the general condition. Studies investigating the characteristics of patients with kidney disease requiring hospitalisation are limited. However, they generally show that admission to nephrology wards is either for diagnostic evaluations or for managing complications[263].

As a result, it is difficult to include these patients in studies or to ask them to complete questionnaires, meaning that the selection of participants from the various hospitals was based on patients who were stable, willing, and in reasonably good condition. The investigators found that these characteristics were more common among outpatients, who either had consultations or underwent chronic hemodialysis sessions.

– Hospital size and type

With regard to bed capacity, the majority of hospitals included in our study were medium sized (75.08 %), 16.83 % were small and were mainly located in East Africa, while only 8.09 % were large and were mainly located in Southern Africa. It is worth noting that one of the main criteria for selecting these hospitals was the availability of one or more nephrologists and specialised care for kidney disease. Additionally, all the selected hospitals were public, given the importance of this healthcare category in the continent. However, they mainly focus on

---

263 Satoshi I, Tetsuji K, Yasuo O et al. Analysis of 2897 hospitalization events for patients with chronic kidney disease: results from CKD-JAC study. *Clinical and Experimental Nephrology* 2019; (23): 956–968.

treating infectious and acute illnesses. Public hospitals are more accessible to the uninsured and the poor than private hospitals, which tends to serve more patients with good health insurance[264].

Previous studies conducted in Africa[265] have found that African patients tended to seek healthcare at public health facilities despite the dissatisfaction of the majority with the services. This paradox can be attributed to their recognition that these public health facilities were staffed by qualified healthcare professionals.

– The replacement therapy for chronic kidney failure

Chronic hemodialysis: The inclusion of chronic hemodialysis patients in our study was easier compared to other patient categories. As a result, 61.5 % of the patients who agreed to participate were chronic hemodialysis patients.

Hemodialysis is a treatment method that acts as a replacement for a failing organ. It is a technique that demands significant human and financial resources and leads to a high level of dependence[266].

Dialysis sessions typically last for 4 to 5 hours, meaning that a hemodialysis patient spends around 12 to 15 hours per week in a healthcare facility – equivalent to the time spent on a full-time job. During these sessions, the patient interacts with caregivers and a complex machine. It is important to recognise that extended absence from these sessions would compromise the patient's life. This vital dependence leads to the development of a special relationship between the nursing staff at the hemodialysis centre and the patient. This unique bond is crucial for providing quality care and could partially explain why many dialysis patients are willing to participate in research and collaborate with the healthcare team to improve overall care management[267].

In our study, 56.1 % of hemodialysis patients underwent 8 hours of dialysis each week, divided into four-hour sessions. Meanwhile, 43.9 % received 12 hours

---

264 Ortiz-Prado E, Ponce J, Cornejo-Leon F et al. Analysis of health and drug access associated with the purchasing power of the Ecuadorian population. *Global Journal of Health Science* 2017; 9(1): 201–210.

265 Health systems in Africa- Community perceptions and perspectives. The report of a multi-country study. World Health Organization, Regional office for Africa: 2012.

266 Pinheiro J. The physician-patient relationship in dialysis. *Portuguese Journal of Nephrology & Hypertension* 2013; 27(3): 179–185.

267 Will T, Saudan P, Droulez MG Et al. Relationship and dependency in a hemodialysis unit. *Néphrologie et thérapeutique* 2008; 4: 320–324.

of dialysis a week, in line with the recommendations of scientific societies. They attended three sessions a week, each lasting four hours.

With the exception of North Africa, where the majority of participants (77.4 % vs. 22.6 %) received the recommended sessions (thrice a week equating to 12 hours), most patients from other African regions in our study only had dialysis twice weekly. Countries where the majority of patients received dialysis thrice weekly included Morocco (73.9 % vs. 26.1 %), Gabon (69.6 % vs. 30.4 %), Tunisia (100 %), Mauritania (60 % vs. 40 %), and Egypt (100 %).

Notably, while national guidelines from most countries recommend thrice weekly therapy, resource constraints in low- and middle-income countries have led to a significant proportion of patients undergoing fewer hemodialysis sessions. This was driven by the need to reduce healthcare costs and enhance dialysis accessibility for more patients in these resource-limited settings[268].

Observational studies[269,270] have shown that patients undergoing hemodialysis twice a week have similar survival rates as those undergoing dialysis thrice a week, provided they follow a strict diet low in protein and potassium to reduce the accumulation of toxins that need to be removed. However, a study conducted in China comparing the health-related quality of life between patients on twice-weekly and thrice-weekly dialysis using the Study Short Form 12 (SF-12) found that the former group had slightly lower scores in physical and mental realms of health-related quality of life, even when adjusted for age and gender differences. Furthermore, patients on the twice-weekly dialysis programme in this study were less likely to have health insurance coverage or a high educational level. The authors recommended randomised controlled trials to better understand the long-term impact of twice-weekly versus thrice-weekly dialysis.

Dialysis consumes a large amount of healthcare resources, making it impossible to provide treatment to all eligible people in most sub-Saharan Africa countries. For instance, in 2010, the estimated number of people in need of dialysis in a year was 19,000 in Kenya, 75,000 in Nigeria, and 6,000 in Senegal. The total cost of hemodialysis was 17 billion USD in Kenya, 35 billion in Nigeria, and 450 million

---

268   Savla D, Chertow GM, Meyer T et al. Can twice weekly hemodialysis expand patient access under resource constraints? *Hemodialysis International* 2017; 21(4): 445–452.
269   Lin YF et al. Comparison of residual renal function in patients undergoing twice-weekly versus three-times-weekly haemodialysis. *Nephrology* 2009; 14: 59–64.
270   Bieber B et al. Two-times weekly hemodialysis in China: frequency, associated patient and treatment characteristics and Quality of Life in the China Dialysis Outcomes and Practice Patterns study. *Nephrology Dialysis Transplantation* 2014; 29: 1770–1777.

in Senegal, which is equivalent to 15 % – 55 % of the total national public health expenditure. The cost of dialysis would consume 8 to 37 % of the total national health expenditure. Studies show that these costs are generally unaffordable for the African states as patients often have to pay out-of-pocket for much of the treatment. Hence, financial constraints strongly influence medical decisions on the number of prescribed hemodialysis sessions. In sub-Saharan Africa, the financial burden means that 59 % of dialysis patients are very often forced to discontinue dialysis despite vital dependence on it.

*Peritoneal dialysis: None of the patients involved in our study underwent peritoneal dialysis, even though this technique is available in some of the targeted countries. A study conducted in France examining the satisfaction of dialysis patients with various techniques (including in-centre hemodialysis, home hemodialysis, and peritoneal dialysis) found that patients were generally satisfied with the care process. Nevertheless, their overall satisfaction was higher for home hemodialysis compared to in-centre hemodialysis (93.3 % vs. 88.4 %), with a higher quality of life noted in home treatment (72.5 % vs. 68.9 %). Furthermore, peritoneal dialysis patients reported higher satisfaction levels compared to home hemodialysis patients (94.4 % vs. 89.7 %)[271].

Barriers to the provision of peritoneal dialysis in many African countries include the rural setting, transportation challenges, low electrification rates, limited access to improved sanitation and water sources, unsuitable living conditions, and a limited number of nephrologists. Cost is a major prohibitive factor due to the price of consumables (dialysis fluids) imported from developed countries. However, local manufacturing of these fluids could greatly facilitate the widespread use of peritoneal dialysis, as demonstrated by the South African example. Additionally, there is an urgent need for education and training of healthcare staff to implement this technique, and international societies can provide valuable assistance in these aspects[272].

Kidney transplantation: In our study, only 2.59 % of patients had a kidney transplant. This accounted for 36.8 % of all Egyptian patients and 6.3 % of all Tunisian patients included in the study. Kidney transplantation is not performed in most African countries, including seven countries involved in our study. As

---

271 Rapport enquête satisfaction patients dialysés. AURAL; 2014.
272 Abu-aisha H, Elamin S. Peritoneal dialysis in Afria. Peritoneal dialysis international: Journal of the International Society for Peritoneal Dialysis. 2010. 30. 23–8.

a result, dialysis is the only treatment option for people with chronic end-stage kidney disease in these countries.

The low number of transplanted patients highlights the challenges surrounding kidney transplantation in Africa. The availability of specialised doctors, surgeons, and laboratories is crucial for making kidney transplantation a viable option for chronic end-stage kidney failure. Moreover, cultural and religious attitudes toward organ donation, trust in the healthcare system and the financial affordability of check-ups, surgery, and anti-rejection immunosuppressive treatments all play significant roles in the realisation of kidney transplantation[273].

Several countries in Africa, including Morocco, Tunisia, Egypt, Sudan, and South Africa, have active living-donor transplantation programmes. However, the practice of transplantation requires significant human and material resources, as well as an appropriate legislative framework. The main barrier to kidney transplantation in Africa is the high cost of transplantation, post-operative care, and particularly the cost of anti-rejection immunosuppressive therapy. Furthermore, many African countries lack government funding, academic support for clinicians, and a proper legislative framework to support transplantation programmes[274].

– Hemodialysis vascular access

In our study, 75.42 % of the chronic haemodialysis patients had a permanent vascular access for hemodialysis, known as the arteriovenous fistula (AVF), while the remaining 24.58 % used a temporary venous catheter for dialysis. In West Africa, the majority of participating patients (69.6 % vs. 30.4 %) used a temporary vascular access. Moreover, 86.7 % of chronic dialysis patients in Senegal relied solely on a temporary vascular access.

Having a permanent and high-quality vascular access (arteriovenous fistula) is crucial for the survival and the well-being of chronic hemodialysis patients. However, in Africa, especially in sub-Saharan Africa, providing this type of vascular access presents a real challenge for dialysis patients. The lack of specialised vascular surgeons, long distances from hospitals that offer this type of surgery, ignorance, and low income often restrict and complicate the implementation and monitoring of these vascular access techniques. Additionally, a significant percentage of patients start their chronic dialysis programme with a temporary

---

273 Muller E. Transplantation in Africa. *Clinical Nephrology* 2016; 86: Suppl. 1 (90–95).
274 Muller E. Transplantation in Africa. *Clinical Nephrology* 2016; 86: Suppl. 1 (90–95).

vascular access option (central venous catheter) due to late referral to the nephrologist, and begin dialysis in an emergency situation.

A study conducted in Senegal revealed that two-thirds of patients underwent their first dialysis using a temporary access, particularly the femoral route, which does not align with the guidelines of professional societies and is associated with a high risk of complications[275].

Furthermore, due to the limited prevalence of hemodialysis in developing countries, including sub-Saharan Africa, there is a scarcity of data regarding vascular access surgery, except in North Africa [276].

Another study on Africa found that 20.65 % of patients started dialysis through a permanent vascular access, while 79.35 % started the dialysis programme using a temporary vascular access (the central venous catheter)[277]. Nwankwo et al.[278] found that, in Nigeria, temporary vascular access was used in 91 % of cases in a cohort of 179 hemodialysis patients over a 5-year period, and in 92.8 % of cases in the Ivory Coast.

It is worth noting that in most sub-Saharan African countries, temporary vascular access is the only available option due to the absence of vascular surgeons, which negatively impacts the quality of dialysis.

7. The patients' perceptions of hospital social responsibility

– Quality and pertinence

We analysed the patients' perceptions of hospitals' social responsibility dimensions based on their satisfaction with : the quality, pertinence, and accessibility of healthcare services as well as the ethical dimension of the care provided.

We examined the participants' perceptions of care quality in three levels: care delivery and treatment effects, the care process, and the hospital's

---

275 Kane Y, Cisse MM, Gaye M, et al. Problematic of vascular access for hemodialysis in sub-Saherienne Africa: experience of Dakar. *Journal of Nephrology & Therapeutics* 2015; 5: 216.
276 Fokou M, Ashuntantang G, Teyang A et al. Patients characteristics and outcome of 518 arterioveinous fistulas for hemodialysis in sub-Saharan African setting. *Annals of Vascular Surgery* 2012; 26: 674–679.
277 Ackoundou-Nguessan C, Gnionsahe A, Guie M et al. High failure rate for first arteriovenous fistula for patients starting hemodialysis treatment: a report from Ivory Coast. *Saudi Journal of Kidney Diseases and Transplantation* 2008; 19: 384e8.
278 Nwankwo EA, Wudiri WW, Bassi A. Practice pattern of hemodialysis vascular access in Maiduguri, Nigeria. *International Journal of Artificial Organs* 2006; 29: 956e60.

overall conditions. Their perception of care pertinence was assessed in two levels: satisfaction with medical prescriptions and check-ups, and satisfaction with anamnesis and doctors' physical examination.

Patients' perceptions of care delivery is increasingly crucial in medical practice. Several methodological studies on hospitals' social responsibility of hospitals focussed on measuring satisfaction with medical care from external stakeholders such as patients.

The success of medical decisions should not only be measured by survival rates, associated comorbidity and tolerability, but also by patients' perceptions of their quality of life and their satisfaction with the care they receive. The impact of the treatment is a crucial indicator of the quality of care. It also helps identify any shortcomings in healthcare programmes and the performance of healthcare staff[279,280].

Treatment involves the use of various healthcare interventions aimed at curing or alleviating disease-related symptoms. Patient satisfaction with treatment refers to their individual evaluation of the process and outcome of the care they receive. Furthermore, it also encompasses their satisfaction with medical care as well as the alignment between their expectations, preferences, and satisfaction with this type of care[281].

In regard to kidney disease, there is limited data on patient satisfaction with the quality and pertinence of care. The kidney patients investigated showed significant differences. Some of the studies were very small, and many of them had questionable reliability and validity[282,283].

Furthermore, commonly used measures of treatment satisfaction, such as attitude response scales, lack precision and are prone to bias, especially when they are single-item. It is also important to consider variations due to language translations, cultural adaptation, and cultural differences. Despite the limitations of the attitude response scales, they offer useful insights into the patient's

---

279   Richardson MM, Paine SS, Grobert ME, Satisfaction with care of patients on hemodialysis. *Clinical Journal of the American Society of Nephrology* 2015; 10(8): 1428–1434.

280   Revicki DA. *Gut* 2004; 53(Suppl IV): iv40–iv44.

281   Weaver M, Patrick DL, Markson LE et al. Issues in the measurement of satisfaction with treatment. *American Journal of Managed Care* 1997; 3: 579–594.

282   Nguyen Thi PL, Frimat L, Loos-Ayav C. SDIALOR: a dialysis patient satisfaction questionnaire. *Néphrologie & Thérapeutique* 2008; 4: 266–277.

283   Morton RL, Tong A, Howard K et al. The views of patients and carers in treatment decision making for chronic kidney disease: systematic review and thematic synthesis of qualitative studies. *BMJ* 2010; 340: c112.

perspective on their current treatment and its effects on the disease. In this study, we used a 5-level closed-ended Likert attitude scale, informally translated into different local dialects, designed for illiterate patients or those who were not fluent in French and English (the original languages of the questionnaire)[284].

Our study revealed that patients from all the African regions and countries included in the study were generally satisfied with the following aspects:

- The treatment effects: 58.4 % of patients were satisfied with the treatment effects, and 30.3 % were very satisfied.
- The doctors' prescriptions: 59 % of patients were satisfied with their doctors' prescriptions, and 31 % were very satisfied.
- The clinical examination: 56.7 % of patients were satisfied with the clinical examination, and 34.9 % were very satisfied.

In multi-centric studies conducted in Western countries, it was found that just under half of hemodialysis patients gave positive feedback on the quality of care[285,286]. Our results are in line with previous Western studies exploring dialysis patients' satisfaction with care, which also indicated that dialysis care was generally satisfactory, especially in terms of treatment effects.

However, the authors of a large multi-centric study[287] conducted in the United States recommended caution in interpreting these results. They noted that patients who followed their doctors' recommendations and clinically stable patients were more likely to participate in surveys assessing their attitudes, perceptions, and experiences of care. In contrast, dissatisfied patients were less likely to take part in such surveys, which may represent a significant selection bias.

Weaver et al.[288] noted that patient factors such as expectations, age, educational level, and personal preferences have an influence on satisfaction with treatment. Moreover, treatment protocols and characteristics such as side

---

284   Revicki DA. *Gut* 2004; 53(Suppl IV): iv40–iv44.
285   Nguyen Thi PL, Frimat L, Loos-Ayav C. SDIALOR: a dialysis patient satisfaction questionnaire. *Néphrologie & Thérapeutique* 2008; 4: 266–277.
286   Morton RL, Tong A, Howard K et al. The views of patients and carers in treatment decision making for chronic kidney disease: systematic review and thematic synthesis of qualitative studies. *BMJ* 2010; 340: c112.
287   Richardson MM, Paine SS, Grobert ME, Satisfaction with care of patients on hemodialysis. *Clinical Journal of the American Society of Nephrology* 2015; 10(8): 1428–1434.
288   Weaver M, Patrick DL, Markson LE et al. Issues in the measurement of satisfaction with treatment. *American Journal of Managed Care* 1997; 3: 579–594.

effects, effectiveness, and the overall healthcare system also affect perceptions of the quality of care received.

It is worth noting that there are several key measurement issues associated with assessing patient perceptions of healthcare quality. The use of attitude response scales and patients' concerns about negative outcomes may skew individual responses and inflate reliability estimates[289,290]. For example, Ross et al.[291] found that favourable responses to satisfaction assessments ranged from 63 % to 82 % depending on the measurement method used. These factors should be considered when interpreting the high satisfaction level among African patients regarding their perceptions of the clinical examination, medical prescriptions and treatment effects.

Regarding questions assessing patient satisfaction with the care process in the hospital—including updates about their disease and treatment, treatment protocols, staff attention, medication side effects and complications—46.8 % of patients were neutral. But generally, patients were less satisfied, with only 29.7 % being satisfied and 19.4 % very satisfied.

It is important to note that while 47.1 % of patients in Southern Africa were satisfied with their hospital care, patients in other African regions were mostly neutral.

At the country level, 38.9 % of Cameroonian patients were either satisfied or very satisfied, while 47.4 % of Egyptian, 50 % of Tunisian, and 47.1 % of Mozambican patients were satisfied. Additionally, 37.1 % of Mauritanian patients were very satisfied. However, patients from other African countries generally remained neutral about the care process. Could this prevailing neutrality be masking a fear of expressing their dissatisfaction, as previously highlighted by other researchers?

It is particularly true when considering the likelihood of dissatisfaction among patients with chronic diseases, such as kidney failure patients, especially those on dialysis. This was observed in a large multicentre study that looked at the satisfaction of hemodialysis patients in Europe and South America[292]. The researchers found that patients were least satisfied with the complex hemodialysis

---

289   Revicki DA. *Gut* 2004; 53(Suppl IV): iv40–iv44.
290   Weaver M, Patrick DL, Markson LE et al. Issues in the measurement of satisfaction with treatment. *American Journal of Managed Care* 1997; 3: 579–594.
291   Ross CK, Steward CA, Sinacore JM. A comparative study of seven measures of patient satisfaction. Medical Care 1995; 33: 392–406.
292   Palmer SC, de Berardis G, Craig JC et al. Patient satisfaction with in-centre haemodialysis care: an international survey. *BMJ Open* 2014; 4: e005020.

care process. However, they were most satisfied with the attention they received from the staff (rated as excellent by 54 % of patients). The least satisfying aspects for them were "information provided when choosing a dialysis modality, prognosis and likelihood of a kidney transplant", "ease of seeing a social worker if needed", and "accuracy of information from a nephrologist". Several Western studies also found dissatisfaction among patients with inadequate information about their therapeutic journey and treatment options[293,294]. Patients expressed a need for more information about the causes and progression of their disease, as well as the symptoms and their impacts. Given that Western patients demand high-quality communication with the medical staff, they perceive inadequate communication as a reflection of misinformation and insensitivity, which is a major concern for them[295,296].

For instance, nearly half of adults with chronic diseases in Norway and Sweden expressed their dissatisfaction with the lack of communication with health professionals regarding their care goals and priorities, condition (in 44 % and 51 % of cases, respectively), or treatment options (52 % and 48 %, respectively). A similar situation was observed in Australia, where one in four adults with chronic diseases did not engage in such discussions with their caregivers[297]. Another notable issue among Western patients with chronic diseases is the coordination of care between different health providers. This often leads to dissatisfaction and becomes a barrier to their overall satisfaction with the care process. Around a third of adults reported encountering at least one of these care coordination problems in Canada, France, Norway, Sweden, Switzerland, and the United States over the past two years. Even in countries scoring with highest scores on this measure, one in five adults continued to report one of

---

293 Ormandy P. Information topics important to chronic kidney disease patients: a systematic review. *Journal of Renal Care* 2008; 34: 19–27.
294 Wachterman M, Marcantonio E, Davis R et al. Relationship between the prognostic expectations of seriously ill patients undergoing hemodialysis and their nephrologists. *JAMA Internal Medicine* 2013; 173: 1206–1214.
295 Palmer SC, de Berardis G, Craig JC et al. Patient satisfaction with in-centre haemodialysis care: an international survey. *BMJ Open* 2014; 4: e005020.
296 Richardson MM, Paine SS, Grobert ME, Satisfaction with Care of Patients on Hemodialysis. *Clinical Journal of the American Society of Nephrology* 2015; 10(8): 1428–1434.
297 Osborn R, Squires D, Doty MM et al. In New survey of eleven countries, US adults still struggle with access to and affordability of health care. *Health Affairs* 2016; 35(12): 2327–2336.

these problems. These findings demonstrate that chronic disease management remains a significant challenge, even in developed countries.

It should be noted that the African patients we targeted in our study did not raise these information, communication, and coordination issues, as they were mostly neutral. In terms of satisfaction with the hospital environment, 45.8 % of the surveyed patients were neutral, 19.7 % were satisfied, 18.1 % were very satisfied, 10.6 % were dissatisfied, and 5.8 % were very dissatisfied across all African regions. Exceptions were noted in Cameroonian patients, who were satisfied with the hospital environment in 38.9 % of cases, and Tunisian patients Cameroonian patients who were satisfied in 43.8 % of cases, while the rest were neutral.

Studies conducted in Western countries indicated that patients with kidney failure, especially those undergoing chronic hemodialysis patients, rated the quality of the hospital environment highly. However, they gave the lowest ratings to the care process, particularly regarding information about treatment options and prognosis, as well as the ease of access to social workers and nephrologists[298,299,300,301].

A study conducted in the United States found that patients good hospital conditions, including cleanliness and a quiet environment, as well as access to information, communication with healthcare providers, quality of nursing services, and pain management, determine the quality of healthcare. Likewise, a study conducted by the WHO in Africa noted that poor infrastructure and the inadequate environment of healthcare facilities contribute to patient dissatisfaction with health services.[302].

Lastly, a study similar to ours conducted in India found that the majority of participating patients were satisfied with the quality of care and performance of

---

298 Palmer SC, de Berardis G, Craig JC et al. Patient satisfaction with in-centre haemodialysis care: an international survey. *BMJ Open* 2014; 4: e005020.
299 Nguyen Thi PL, Frimat L, Loos-Ayav C. SDIALOR: A dialysis patient satisfaction questionnaire. *Néphrologie & Thérapeutique* 2008; 4: 266–277.
300 Ormandy P. Information topics important to chronic kidney disease patients: a systematic review. *Journal of Renal Care* 2008; 34: 19–27.
301 Wachterman M, Marcantonio E, Davis R et al. Relationship between the prognostic expectations of seriously ill patients undergoing hemodialysis and their nephrologists. *JAMA Internal Medicine* 2013; 173: 1206–1214.
302 Health systems in Africa- Community perceptions and perspectives. The report of a multi-country study. World Health Organization, Regional office for Africa: 2012.

their doctors. However, they complained about the poor conditions in which healthcare was provided[303].

– Access to healthcare

In terms of "access", 46.6 % of patients were neutral about their satisfaction with waiting times for consultation or hospitalisation, 19.4 % were satisfied and 17.2 % very satisfied. On the other hand, 10 % of patients were dissatisfied or very dissatisfied in 6.8 % of cases. In contrast to Southern Africa, where 47.1 % of patients were satisfied with healthcare waiting times, patients from other African regions were generally neutral.

44.4 % of patients in Cameroon were very satisfied with waiting times. 47.1 % of patients in Mozambique and 56.3 % Tunisia were satisfied. Patients from other countries were generally neutral about waiting times.

An American and European multicentric study[304] exploring how hemodialysis patients perceived care found that accessibility of care and ease of reaching staff received excellent ratings.

Regarding the availability of medicines at the hospital level, the study found that 41.7 % of patients were neutral, 21.8 % were satisfied, and 11.7 % were very satisfied. In contrast, 15.3 % of patients were dissatisfied and 9.4 % very dissatisfied. Notably, except for Central Africa where 38.8 % of patients were satisfied, and West Africa, where 29.8 % of patients were very dissatisfied with the availability of free-of-cost medicines in their hospitals, the majority of patients from other regions were neutral. 38.9 % of the surveyed patients from Cameroon, 66.6 % from Gabon, and 43.8 % from Chad were satisfied with the availability of free-of-cost medicines in their hospitals. In Senegal, 53.3 % of patients were satisfied, and 46.7 % very dissatisfied. Patients from other countries were generally neutral about this issue.

As for patient satisfaction with the overall healthcare costs (including treatment, laboratory tests, and medical imaging), 45.1 % of patients were neutral, 16.2 % were satisfied, and 18.5 % were very satisfied. On the other hand, 15.3 % were dissatisfied, and 4.9 % were very dissatisfied. Except for Southern Africa, where 41.2 % of patients were satisfied with the treatment costs, patients from other regions were generally neutral. 32.7 % of Moroccan patients were dissatisfied, while 40 % of Senegalese patients were very satisfied. Moreover,

---

303 Nirupam M. Attitudes and perceptions of medical doctors towards their jobs in the state of J&K, India. *International Journal of Health* 2007; 1(2).

304 Palmer SC, de Berardis G, Craig JC et al. Patient satisfaction with in-centre haemodialysis care: an international survey. *BMJ Open* 2014; 4: e005020.

41.2 % of Mozambican patients and 34.5 % of Gabonese patients were satisfied. Finally, patients from other countries were broadly neutral about this issue.

The lack of access to healthcare was crystal clear from a multicentric study conducted by the WHO in the African region[305]. The main reasons behind patients' negative perceptions of public health facilities were the lack of medications, unfriendliness of healthcare providers, and long waiting times. Conversely, satisfied patients highlighted responsiveness of healthcare providers and the good environment as the main factors behind their satisfaction[306,307,308]. In fact, according to the WHO study, the main barriers to healthcare access were the healthcare costs, long travel distances to health facilities, inadequate and unaffordable transport systems, low quality of healthcare, and unfriendliness of healthcare providers. For instance, when implementing the African Programme for Onchocerciasis Control (APOC) in the Democratic Republic of Congo, it was found that 20 % of onchocerciasis endemic communities were located 11 to 20 kilometres from the nearest healthcare facility. Additionally, the lack of qualified healthcare professionals, discrimination against patients unable to pay for health services and poor organisation were found to be major challenges to healthcare access[309,310,311,312].

---

305 Health systems in Africa- Community perceptions and perspectives. The report of a multi-country study. World Health Organization, Regional office for Africa: 2012.
306 Swanson RC et al. Toward a consensus on guiding principles for health systems strengthening. *PLoS Med* 2010; 7(12): e1000385.
307 Addendum for the plan of action and budget 2008–2012. World Health Organization and African Programme for Onchocerciasis Control (APOC). WHO; 2008. Available at: <https://apps.who.int/iris/handle/10665/274421/browse?authority=Strategic+Planning&type=mesh>.
308 Revicki, D. A., Gut 2004; 53 (Suppl IV): iv40–iv44.
309 Dechambenoit G. Access to health care in sub-Saharan Africa. *Surgical Neurology International* 2016; 7:108.
310 Swanson RC et al. Toward a consensus on guiding principles for health systems strengthening. *PLoS Med* 2010; 7(12): e1000385.
311 Closing the gap in health equity through action on the social determinants of health. Geneva: World Health Organization Commission on Social Determinants on Health. WHO; 2008. Available at: <http://www.who.int/social_determinants/thecommission/finalre-port/en/index.html>.
312 Addendum for the plan of action and budget 2008–2012. World Health Organization and African Programme for Onchocerciasis Control (APOC). WHO; 2008. Available at: <https://apps.who.int/iris/handle/10665/274421/browse?authority=Strategic+Planning&type=mesh>.

It is important to note that access to healthcare is a widespread issue worldwide, with less severity in developed countries than in Africa. In a survey conducted in eleven developed countries – Australia, Canada, France, Germany, the Netherlands, New Zealand, Norway, Sweden, Switzerland, the United Kingdom, and the United States – some patients reported their inability to see a doctor or nurse when needed, neither on the same day nor on the following day. About half of Canadian, German, and Norwegian adults (47–53 %) could not get an appointment on the first two days of the disease. At least one in five patients in Canada, Germany, Norway, Sweden, and the United States had to wait six days or more. On the other hand, only one in five adults in the Netherlands and New Zealand managed to see a health professional on the same day or the following day[313].

Emergency departments often serve as the default healthcare provider. One-third or more of adults in Canada, France, Sweden, and the United States reported visiting the emergency departments in the past two years. In Canada, where accessing primary care has been an issue, (30 %) of adults reported waiting two months or more before seeing a specialist, followed by Norwegian adults (28 %). In contrast, less than 10 % of patients in France, Germany, the Netherlands, Switzerland, and the United States reported waiting that long.

The lack of medicines and patient dissatisfaction with treatment costs can be attributed to the fact that very few African countries have met the target of allocating 15 % of their GDP to improving the health sector (Abuja Declaration, 2001). When 60–70 % of hospital resources are spent on salaries and staff expenses, there is little left for other costs[314,315]. Adding to this, sub-Saharan governments had to comply with structural adjustment policies recommended by the World Bank and the International Monetary Fund (IMF). As a consequence, in poorer countries, people are more likely to pay out-of-pocket for healthcare. This flawed system has been criticised by Joseph Stiglitz, Nobel Prize winner in economics (2001) and former World Bank chief economist[316].

---

313 Osborn R, Squires D, Doty MM et al. In New survey of eleven countries, US adults still struggle with access to and affordability of health care. *Health Affairs* 2016; 35(12): 2327–2336.
314 Dechambenoit G. Access to health care in sub-Saharan Africa. *Surgical Neurology International* 2016; 7: 108.
315 Brunet-Jailly. *Innover dans les systèmes de santé; expériences d' Afrique de l'Ouest.* Paris: Karthala, 1997: 257–270.
316 Stiglitz J. *Globalization and its discontents.* Fayard: Paris; 2002.

In wealthier countries, per capita health expenditure is around 3,100 USD, while in sub-Saharan Africa it is estimated at 37 USD[317].

On the other hand, according to the WHO study, African patients saw the lack of medicines as contributing to the negative perceptions around the quality of care in healthcare facilities. This explains the prevalence of self-medication, ineffective alternatives, and the frequent use of traditional healers in African communities, further delaying necessary medical care and impacting patient prognosis. Moreover, the research findings indicated that African patients often had difficulty obtaining the prescribed medications because they were either non-available or unaffordable. The findings also highlighted the overall shortage of medical supplies in the surveyed healthcare facilities[318]. These examples indicate that the lack of access to healthcare has significant medical and social implications. It can lead to the deterioration of people's health and the loss of confidence in the healthcare system.

– Professional ethics

Medical practice requires a high level of ethical standards. The ethical conduct that should govern the doctor-patient relationship should include respecting patients' autonomy, which involves giving them control over decisions about their health. It also includes respecting their privacy, and providing care in an equitable manner and in line with current scientific knowledge. Therefore, our study focussed on the ethical aspects of the medical profession by examining factors such as equal access to healthcare, the opportunity for treatment regardless of the patients' financial status, and the protection of patient privacy.

Regarding the perception of equity in access to healthcare at the hospital, 49 % of patients were neutral, 22.1 % were satisfied, and 23.4 % were very satisfied. Only 5.5 % of patients expressed dissatisfaction. Satisfaction levels varied across different African regions. For example, 32.7 % of patients from West Africa were satisfied, while patients from other African regions tended to be more neutral. 38.9 % of Cameroonian patients, 41.6 % of Moroccan patients, and 41.2 % of Mauritanian patients were very satisfied. Additionally, 41.2 of Mozambican patients and 68.8 % of Tunisian patients were satisfied. Most patients from other countries were neutral about this issue.

---

317   World development indicators. World Bank; 2020. Available at: <http: //data.worldb ank.org/indicator/SH>. XPD . PC AP .

318   Health systems in Africa- Community perceptions and perspectives. The report of a multi-country study. World Health Organization, Regional office for Africa: 2012.

As for access to care regardless of the ability to pay, 49.8 % of patients said it was only sometimes possible, 23.6 % said it was usually possible, 6.9 % said it was only rarely possible, and 3.6 % said it was never possible.

In Southern Africa, 41.2 % of participating patients indicated that they could usually receive care regardless of their ability to pay. However, patients from other parts of the continent reported that this was only "sometimes possible".

33.3 % of Cameroonian patients and 41.2 % of Mozambican patients stated that they were usually able to receive treatment regardless of their ability to pay, while the majority of patients in other countries expressed a neutral stance on this issue.

In the multicentric study conducted by the WHO in Africa[319], some patients expressed concerns about the unequal distribution of health services by the government. Overall, 40.5 % of the respondents stated they were still confident in the public healthcare system's ability to meet their needs. About 41.1 % of the respondents stated they were sometimes confident in the government's ability to provide health services properly. However, 13.8 % stated they never trusted the government to act properly and fairly in the people's best interest. It is worth noting that patients from rural areas, who reported always trusting the government to provide good and fair care, were more numerous than those from urban areas.

Distrust of public hospitals in terms of equity is partly due to the persistent shortage of medicines and health staff, high treatment costs as well, and negative attitudes of health workers towards patients, especially the most vulnerable who cannot afford healthcare. This type of distrustful attitude towards healthcare facilities and the associated negative perception of them as being unequal is much less common in European countries. According to the WHO, equity in healthcare is closely related to the implementation of universal health coverage. The latter means that all people have access to the full range of quality health services they need – including prevention, promotion, treatment, rehabilitation, and palliative care, without the risk of financial hardship from paying such services. This requires a robust, efficient, and well-managed healthcare system that enables all people to access good quality services, health workers, medicines, and technologies. It also requires a financing system to protect people from financial hardship and impoverishment from healthcare costs. The WHO highlights that "access to health services ensures healthier people; while financial risk protection prevents people from being pushed into poverty. Therefore,

---

319 Health systems in Africa- Community perceptions and perspectives. The report of a multi-country study. World Health Organization, Regional office for Africa: 2012.

universal health coverage is a critical component of sustainable development and poverty reduction, and a key element to reducing social inequities"[320].

An efficient and equitable healthcare system is one that addresses priority health needs through integrated, person-centred care. This involves information and awareness campaigns, as well as accessible and affordable preventive, curative, and rehabilitative care. It requires an adequate number of qualified healthcare professionals, as well as a sufficient supply of medicines, diagnostic and treatment equipment. Addressing the social determinants of health such as education, living conditions, and income is also crucial for improving people's health and access to healthcare services.

Regarding patients' satisfaction with the measures taken to protect their privacy, 47.9 % were neutral, 30.6 % were satisfied, 18.6 % were very satisfied, and 3 % were dissatisfied.

In West Africa, 44.9 % of participating patients were satisfied with the privacy measures, while patients from other African regions were generally neutral. 77.8 % of Cameroonian patients, 47.1 % of Mauritanian patients, and 75 % of Tunisian patients were satisfied. Patients from other countries were generally neutral about this.

The patient's right to privacy entails keeping patient information confidential. From a historical perspective, legal documents related to patients' rights have consistently emphasised the importance of privacy and confidentiality. Examples include the Patients' Bill of Rights of the American Hospital Association in 1972, the Amsterdam Declaration on the Promotion of Patients' Rights in Europe in 1994, and the European Charter of Patients' Rights in 2002. Confidentiality and privacy are crucial for building and maintaining an effective and respectful clinical relationship. Respecting patient privacy means that doctors must keep information shared by patients or obtained during professional interactions confidential. Privacy is also a social benefit because it allows for open discussions of health issues between patients and clinicians in a safe and trusted environment[321].

There have been limited studies in Africa that aimed to determine the extent of privacy and personal data protection[322]. Questions have also been raised as to

---

320   Questions and Answers on Universal Health Coverage. World Health Organization; 2020. Available at: <https://www.who.int/healthsystems/topics/financing/uhc_qa/en/>.
321   Demirsoy N, Kirimlioglu N. Protection of privacy and confidentiality as a patient right: physicians' and nurses' viewpoints. *Biomedical Research* 2016; 27(4).
322   Townsend BA. Privacy and data protection ehealth in Africa (PhD thesis). South Africa: Univ. of Cape Town; 2017.

whether the Westernised notion of privacy aligns with the traditional African view or if it is mainly a Western issue.

Before the 1960s and 1970s, Africa had few to no data protection policies. At that time, technological and informational developments were limited on the continent, and regulations were not relevant. However, in the following years, especially with the widespread introduction of the digital age, new privacy issues emerged. These issues were driven by the urge to strengthen protection in a rapidly evolving global digital environment. As a result, privacy measures began to receive due consideration. Many authors hold that African values are less about privacy and individualism and more about the collective good. However, there is likely to be a change in the perception of the value of privacy in Africa, as evidenced by the emergence of recent data protection laws[323].

Privacy is considered a human right, but there are cultural differences in how privacy is understood within and across regions. Defining privacy is challenging because of its complex nature. Adding to this difficulty is the relatively recent recognition of human rights compared to traditional laws in Africa and the East. The presence of data protection laws in Africa, as well as the lack of agreement between nations, has led to varying cross-border rules and procedures, creating privacy landscape. Many African countries are still in the process of establishing their Many African data protection systems, and regulations remain either on paper or are progressing slowly. Furthermore, there are significant gaps in the literature on data protection and privacy issues in many parts of Africa, with some issues being under-researched or not researched at all.

An American study[324] focussing on patients' perspectives of medical confidentiality in hospitals found that many patients were unaware of or misunderstood their legal or ethical right to medical confidentiality protections. The possibility that medical information might be revealed, intentionally or not, troubles patients. A significant minority of patients distrust confidentiality protections, leading some to report that they delay or forgo medical care. In addition, this study revealed a wide variety of understandings and beliefs about medical confidentiality among patients, which are often not indicated in the writings of practitioners or legal experts. As medical confidentiality regulations evolve, these differences need to be recognised and accounted for in interactions between practitioners and patients.

---

323 Townsend BA. Privacy and Data protection ehealth in Africa (PhD thesis). South Africa: Univ. of Cape Town; 2017.

324 Sankar P, Mora S, Merz J et al. Patient perspectives of medical confidentiality: a review of the literature. *Journal of General Internal Medicine* 2003; 18: 659–669.

It is important to recognise the potential dangers associated with disregarding patient privacy. When information is disclosed, it can negatively affects individuals' well-being by compromising their ability to secure a job, obtain insurance, or hold positions of responsibility. Additionally, safeguarding health information helps individuals avoid the social stigma often linked to certain health conditions.

There is limited data on how kidney patients, especially those from Africa, perceive confidentiality. Given this situation, neutral responses may be seen as hidden dissatisfaction or a lack of understanding regarding the importance of this issue[325,326]

– Patients' perceptions of hospital social responsibility

49.35 % of patients gave an average rating of the social responsibility of their hospitals, while 26.95 % perceived it as good, and 12.66 % considered it poor. In Southern Africa, 76.5 % of patients rated their hospitals' as good, while patients from other regions generally rated it as average. 65.5 % of patients from Gabon, 76.5 % from Mozambique, and 46.7 % from Senegal rated their hospitals' social responsibility as good. Patients from other countries generally considered it as average (figure 12).

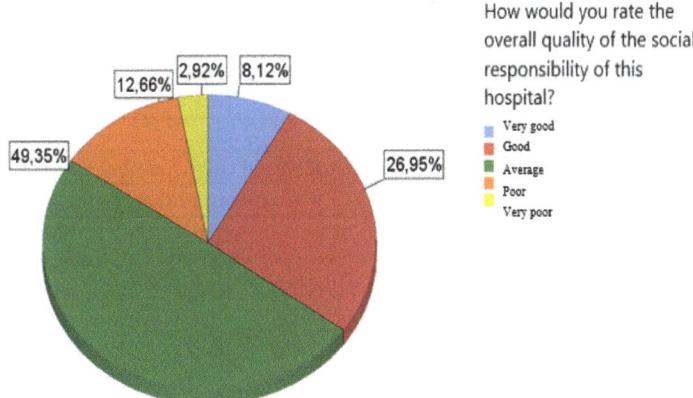

Figure 12: Patients' perceptions of hospital social responsibility

---

325 Demirsoy N, Kirimlioglu N. Protection of privacy and confidentiality as a patient right: physicians' and nurses' viewpoints. *Biomedical Research* 2016; 27(4).
326 McGraw D, Greene SM, Miner CS et al. Privacy and confidentiality in pragmatic clinical trials. *Clinical Trials* 2015; 12(5): 520–529.

In a 2016 study conducted in China[327], the majority of patients were either satisfied or very satisfied with the social responsibility of the surveyed public hospitals. With the exception of "the provision of treatment regardless of ability to pay", all other aspects received high scores. This differs from the findings of our study revealing that patients were generally satisfied with their nephrologists' prescriptions, treatment effectiveness, and the care process. However, the hospital environment, waiting times, overall treatment, and availability of medicines and medical tests were perceived as unsatisfactory. Additionally, most of our patients thought that receiving treatment regardless of their ability to pay is not always possible.

The Chinese study also found that the way hospitals provide care can impact how patients perceive hospital social responsibility. The study revealed that the "service quality", "pertinence", "accessibility", and "professional ethics" scores were positively linked to patients' views of hospital social responsibility.

In our survey, the multi-level linear regression analysis of patients' perceptions of hospital social responsibility showed that neither patients' characteristics nor "service quality" and "pertinence" were associated with their perceptions. However, an "accessibility"-related item (cost of treatment p: -0.003) was negatively associated, while a "professional ethics"-related item (privacy p:0.039) was positively associated (Table 6).

Table 6: Multi-level linear regression models of patients' overall assessment of hospital social responsibility

Coefficients [a]			
	Non-standardised coefficients		p
	A	Standard error	
Gender	-,205	,116	,081
Age	-,001	,004	,781
Type of patient	,250	,128	,053
Health coverage	,168	,121	,164
Educational level	,100	,064	,117
Income	,044	,099	,657

---

327 Liu W, Shi L, Pong RW et al. How patients think about social responsibility of public hospitals in China?. *BMC Health Services Research* 2016; 16: 371.

Table 6: Fortsetzung

Coefficients ª			
Quality:	,057	,091	,536
Satisfaction with the provision and effects of the treatment	-,125,023	,079	,115
Satisfaction with the care process		,063	,713
Satisfaction with the environment and the general conditions			
Pertinence:	,152	,110,094	,169
Satisfaction with the medical prescriptions	-,002		,982
Satisfaction with the anamnesis and the clinical examination			
Accessibility:	,001	,063	,983
Satisfaction with the waiting times	,182	,060	-,003
Satisfaction with the costs of treatment	-,036	,065	,580
Availability of medicines in the hospital			
Professional ethics:	-,177	,085	,039
Satisfaction with privacy protection measures	-,056	,069	,420
Satisfaction with equitable access to health care			

a. Dependent variable: The perception of hospital social responsibility

Schermerhorn[328] and Kurniawan[329] noted that CSR involves four main levels of action: profitability, legitimacy, ethics, and philanthropy. These four elements can be grouped into two categories: the first concerns the legal obligations of the organisation in question, while the second involves voluntary actions. Hospital social responsibility is a broad concept, encompassing not only healthcare but also other activities such as training paramedical teams, conducting health seminars, providing counselling, engaging in philanthropy, and participating in environmental activities. These activities can significantly impact the hospital's

---

328 Schermerhorn JR. *Management*. 6th Asia-Pacific ed. Melbourne: Wiley; 2016.
329 Kurniawan R. Effect of environmental performance on environmental disclosures of manufacturing, mining and plantation companies listed in Indonesia stock exchange. Arthatama: *Journal of Business Management and Accounting* 2017; 1(1): 6–17.

value and reputation, enhance its brand image, and foster long-term patient loyalty. Our study specifically focusses on the perceptions of CSR and its dimensions in relation to people's health and services.

In the healthcare context, Bosho and Gray[330], Wu[331], and Naidu[332] found that the assurance and quality of patient care provided by healthcare staff have a positive impact on patient satisfaction, patient loyalty, and patients' perceptions of their hospital's social responsibility. Healthcare providers must offer high-quality service and maintain excellent hygiene standards. According to Meyer et al.[333], patients pay close attention to hospital services and quality, especially the success rate and failure rates of treatments.

A study conducted in Indonesia[334] looked into how patients perceived the social responsibility of hospitals. It found that they generally rated the social responsibility of public hospitals as relatively good. However, there was wide range of responses, as some patients perceived it as very good, while others did not. The assessment was based on three main aspects related to hospital services: quality, pertinence, and the financial aspect.

It is also important to consider the perspectives that highlight the direct, negative impact of social responsibility on the value of hospitals. This occurs when relatively high additional costs are imposed on patients, despite the potential benefits of such measure. These benefits include increased levels of service efficiency and pertinence, as well as improved financial performance of the hospital thanks to more qualified medical staff. Supporters of this view pointed to the inefficient use of service time and staff resources, "waste" of operating funds, and inefficient patient scheduling, which can seriously affect the hospital's reputation and patient loyalty.

---

330 Bosho C, Gray B. The relationships between service quality, customer satisfaction and buying intentions in the private hospital industry. *South African Journal of Business Management* 2004; 35(4): 27–37.
331 Wu CC. The impact of hospital brand image on service quality, patient satisfaction and loyalty. *African Journal of Business Management* 2011; 5(12): 4873.
332 Naidu A. Factors affecting patient satisfaction and healthcare quality. *International Journal of Health Care Quality Assurance* 2009; 22(4): 366–381.
333 Meyer JA, Silow-Carroll S, Stepnick LS et al. Hospital quality: ingredients for success – overview and lessons learned. New York, NY: The Commonwealth Fund; 2004.
334 Lubis AN. Corporate social responsibility in health sector: a case study in the government hospitals in Medan, Indonesia. *Verslas: Teorija Ir Praktika / Business: Theory and practice* 2018; 19: 25–36.

The factors mentioned above were not observed in our patients as they did not have multiple hospital options to choose from, nor did they have the option to be loyal or not.

- Correlations between patients' socio-demographic data and their perceptions of hospital social responsibility

We hypothesised that the patients' perceptions of hospital social responsibility, as determined by the survey items, might be related to their socio-demographic characteristics.

Our analysis of the correlations between patients' socio-demographic data and their perceptions of hospitals' social responsibility demonstrated statistically significant differences in the following areas:

- African region: Patients from Southern and Central Africa participating in this study had a more positive perception of hospital social responsibility (p:0.000, IC:95 %).
- Hospital size: Patients treated in larger hospitals were more satisfied (p: 0.002, IC:95 %).
- Place of residence: Urban patients were less satisfied than rural patients (p:0.015, IC:95 %).
- Patient type: Inpatients were more satisfied than outpatients (p: 0.04, CI:95 %).
- Health coverage: Patients with health coverage were more satisfied (p: 0.0448, CI: 95 %).

However, statistical analysis showed no significant correlation between patients' perceptions of hospital social responsibility and other parameters such as age, gender, income, or educational level (Table 7).

Table 7: Correlations between patients' sociodemographic data and their perceptions of hospital social responsibility

		Perception of hospital social responsibility			P
		Good	Average	Bad	
Region	Southern Africa	76,5 %	23,5 %	0 %	,0000
	Central Africa	46,8 %	39,2 %	13,9 %	
	East Africa	0 %	81,5 %	18,5 %	
	West Africa	22,4 %	63,3 %	14,3 %	
	North Africa	34,6 %	47,1 %	18,4 %	

(fortgeführt)

Table 7: Fortsetzung

		Perception of hospital social responsibility			P
Hospital size	Large > 500 beds	68,0 %	28,0 %	4,0 %	,002
	Average: 100– 500 beds	34,6 %	49,8 %	15,6 %	
	Small <100 beds	21,6 %	56,9 %	21,6 %	
Gender	Male	33,7 %	51,4 %	14,9 %	,690
	Female	36,8 %	46,4 %	16,8 %	
Patient type	Inpatient	42,9 %	50,0 %	7,1 %	,040
	Outpatient (for consultation or for dialysis)	30,3 %	49,0 %	20,7 %	
Place of residence	Urban	35,2 %	47,7 %	17,1 %	,015
	Rural	36,5 %	59,5 %	4,1 %	
Health coverage	Yes	37,8 %	49,4 %	12,8 %	,0448
	No	30,3 %	54,5 %	15,2 %	
Educational level	None	36,4 %	57,6 %	6,1 %	0,30
	Primary	24,2 %	62,9 %	12,9 %	
	Secondary	37,0 %	41,3 %	21,7 %	
	Tertiary	39,4 %	43,7 %	16,9 %	
Income	Low	33,3 %	53,3 %	13,3 %	0,198
	Average	33,1 %	46,5 %	20,5 %	
	High	50,0 %	36,7 %	13,3 %	
Age (in years)	0–18	0 %	100,0 %	0 %	0,312
	18–25	27,8 %	66,7 %	5,6 %	
	25–35	31,5 %	51,9 %	16,7 %	
	35–45	35,5 %	50,0 %	14,5 %	
	45–55	43,8 %	43,8 %	12,3 %	
	55–65	27,9 %	52,5 %	19,7 %	
	65–75	45,0 %	30,0 %	25,0 %	
	75–85	37,5 %	62,5 %	0 %	

In contrast to our findings, a study on French dialysis patients found that their satisfaction was largely influenced by age, as older patients were more satisfied than younger ones. Gender or place of residence did not seem to have an impact on satisfaction scores[335].

---

335 Nguyen Thi PL, Frimat L, Loos-Ayav C. SDIALOR: A dialysis patient satisfaction questionnaire. *Néphrologie & Thérapeutique* 2008; 4: 266–277.

Additionally, Palmer et al.[336] discovered in a multicentric study of European and South American hemodialysis patients that older respondents tended to give higher scores to overall care. Similar trends were observed in studies examining patient satisfaction across various healthcare services.

Moreover, a previous WHO study on healthcare systems in Africa[337] revealed that over two-thirds of patients were dissatisfied with public healthcare. The overall dissatisfaction rate was 64.3 %, with breakdowns by residence as follows: urban-66.7 %, peri-urban-62.7 %, and rural-64.6 %. However, a study[338] analysing the satisfaction of Saudi patients with public healthcare facilities indicated that women were less satisfied with the services compared to men, whose satisfaction was considered significant.

In addition, the Saudi authors found a strong correlation between higher levels of education and better satisfaction rates. They also noted that patients satisfied with their income level were generally satisfied with the health services provided by the hospital. Dissatisfied patients attributed their dissatisfaction mainly to the unclear explanation of disease-related and medicine-related information by the healthcare providers, possibly due to the language barrier. The educational level and income were not associated with patient perceptions in our survey. Similar to our study, the authors found no other significant association between the satisfaction with healthcare facilities and age.

In 2016, a survey[339] of eleven countries – Australia, Canada, France, Germany, the Netherlands, New Zealand, Norway, Sweden, Switzerland, the United Kingdom, and the United States – found that financial barriers hindered access to healthcare in developed countries. The access varied considerably between countries, reflecting differences in health insurance design, organisation, and the capacity of essential care services. Countries may excel in health insurance but lag in organisation and essential care capacity. Unless adults show strong performance in both areas, a substantial number of them will find it difficult

---

336   Palmer SC, de Berardis G, Craig JC et al. Patient satisfaction with in-centre haemodialysis care: an international survey. *BMJ Open* 2014; 4: e005020.
337   Health systems in Africa- Community perceptions and perspectives. The report of a multi-country study. World Health Organization, Regional office for Africa: 2012.
338   Almutairi OO, Alqarni AA, Alzahrani SA et al. Patients' satisfaction with health care services in Southern Saudi Arabia. *The Egyptian Journal of Hospital Medicine* 2018; 72(1): 3857–3860.
339   Osborn R, Squires D, Doty MM et al. In New survey of eleven countries, US adults still struggle with access to and affordability of health care. *Health Affairs* 2016; 35(12): 2327–2336.

to obtain health care. The study revealed that American adults were the most likely to report financial barriers to healthcare, with 33 % reporting a cost-related access problem in the year prior to the study. Swiss adults were the second most likely to report such barriers. On the other hand, only 7–8 % of adults in Germany, the Netherlands, Sweden, and the UK reported being unable to afford necessary medical care.

In all the surveyed countries, low-income adults were much more likely to report experiencing health and financial issues than others. As a result, their experience with healthcare reflected how well their country's healthcare system was meeting the needs of its most socially vulnerable patients. In the United States, 43 % of low-income adults reported cost-related barriers to healthcare access, representing the highest percentage among all the surveyed countries. The UK was the only country where low-income adults were less likely to report cost-related problems compared to the rest of the population. In Canada, France, Germany, Sweden, the United Kingdom, and the United States, low-income adults reported longer waiting times for healthcare than the rest of the population. In these countries, one third or more reported having to wait at least six days to see a health professional. Additionally, between a quarter and a half of low-income adults in most countries reported using the emergency service in the last two years, possibly due to the lack of timely access to healthcare, thus explaining their dissatisfaction with healthcare services. Such data highlights the numerous unresolved challenges affecting the provision of care for this population segment, even in industrialised countries whose primary goal is to provide accessible, affordable, and high-quality healthcare.

Our study unexpectedly did not find a link between income level and the perception of hospital social responsibility. However, we did find that having health coverage was highly and significantly associated with our patients' satisfaction. Several previous studies have also found that healthcare systems with universal health coverage are better at removing financial barriers to healthcare access, which was positively seen by patients[340,341]. Additionally,

---

340 Osborn R, Squires D, Doty MM et al. In New survey of eleven countries, US adults still struggle with access to and affordability of health care. *Health Affairs* 2016; 35(12): 2327–2336.
341 Fenton JJ; Jerant AF; Bertakis KD. The cost of satisfaction a national study of patient satisfaction. Health care utilization, expenditures, and mortality. *Arch Intern Med* 2012; 172(5): 405–411.

in line with our findings, a study conducted in the United Stated[342] found no significant difference in patient satisfaction between university hospitals and other healthcare facilities. The authors of this study also noted that patients in small hospitals were more satisfied than those in large hospitals.

Notably, an earlier study[343] conducted in Ghana showed that individuals living in communities with larger health facilities tended to be healthier and more satisfied due to the increased availability of medical supplies. The same result was found in our study.

- Correlations between countries' socio-economic data and patients' perception of hospital social responsibility

Our analysis of statistical correlations between countries' socio-economic data and patients' perceptions of hospital social responsibility revealed a significant positive association between country's income (p:0.000), health expenditure (PPP USD) (p:0.011), and public expenditure on education (% GDP) (p:0.000) on the one hand, and perceived hospital social responsibility on the other hand.

The findings of our study align with numerous other well-conducted studies indicating a strong positive correlation between patient satisfaction and public health expenditure. This expenditure is closely linked to the income level of a country. A patient from a high-income country is about 3400 times more likely to be satisfied with their country's healthcare system than a patient from a low-income country. This disparity between "high income" and "low income" countries reflects the different perceptions among patients from different economic backgrounds. For example, patients in wealthier countries tend to be more satisfied with the healthcare system than those in other economies (Table 8).

---

342 Ashish K. Jha E. Orav J et al. Patients' perception of hospital care in the United States. *The New England Journal of Medicine* 2008; 359: 1921–1931.
343 Lavy V, Strauss J, Duncan Thomas et al. Quality of health care, survival and health outcomes in Ghana. *Journal of Health Economics* 1996; 15: 333–357.

Table 8: Correlations between countries' socio-economic data and patients' perceptions of hospital social responsibility

		Perceptions of hospital social responsibility			p
		Good	Average	Bad	
Country's income	Upper middle	72,4 %	17,2 %	10,3 %	0,000
	Lower middle	30,5 %	50,7 %	18,7 %	
	Lower	32,9 %	57,9 %	9,2 %	
	Total	35,1 %	49,4 %	15,6 %	
Per capita health expenditure (PPP USD)	<100	32,9 %	57,9 %	9,2 %	0,011
	100–300	22,4 %	58,2 %	19,4 %	
	300–500	40,6 %	37,6 %	21,8 %	
	500–700	47,9 %	45,8 %	6,3 %	
	700–800	25,0 %	56,3 %	18,8 %	
	Total	35,1 %	49,4 %	15,6 %	
Public health expenditure (in % GDP)	<5 %	24,4 %	62,2 %	13,4 %	0,000
	5–10 %	43,6 %	36,9 %	19,5 %	
	>10 %	37,5 %	56,3 %	6,3 %	
	Total	35,1 %	49,4 %	15,6 %	

Chapter 3: Nephrologists: The characteristics and perceptions of hospital social responsibility

Nephrology is a relatively new field, initially established as a separate subspecialty in Europe in 1949 and in the United States in the 1960s. The global capacity for nephrology training and professionals remains largely unknown. According to a multinational survey conducted by the International Society of Nephrology (ISN), the global density of nephrologists was 8.83 per million population (pmp). High-income countries reported a nephrologist density of 28.52 pmp, compared to 0.31 pmp in low-income countries[344].

Indeed, the survey revealed significant differences in the global distribution of nephrologists and nephrology trainees, indicating an overall shortage of all healthcare providers in nephrology. This shortage was particularly pronounced in low-income countries, especially in the African and South Asian regions.

Out of the ten countries with the lowest density of nephrologists, nine are located in Africa, namely in sub-Saharan Africa. The lowest density was reported in Malawi (0.06 pmp), Mozambique (0.08 pmp), and Ethiopia (0.09 pmp). On the other hand, the highest density was reported in North African countries such as Egypt (21.65 pmp), Tunisia (16.31 pmp), Libya (12.48 pmp), and Algeria (11.38 pmp). In North Africa, the density of nephrologists in Tunisia and Egypt was above 15 per million population, and between 10.1 and 15 in Morocco. The density of nephrologists in countries belonging to other regions was less than 5 pmp. These countries include Mauritania, Senegal, Cameroon, Chad, Burundi, and Mozambique.

African nephrology, like other medical fields, is experiencing a significant brain drain. Many doctors and scientists who leave Africa for training abroad never return to their home country[345]. Research has shown that this shortage of doctors, particularly specialists, has serious repercussions on African populations, such as delayed referral to nephrologists, challenges in managing kidney disease, and other impacts. It is also worth pointing to a study[346] which

---

344 Osman MA et al. Health workforce for nephrology care: existing manpower and training capacity. *Kidney International Supplements* 2018; 8: 52–63.
345 Swanepoel CR, Wearne N, Okpechi IG. Nephrology in Africa – not yet uhuru. *Nature Reviews Nephrology* 2013 Oct; 9(10): 610–622.
346 Lavy V, Strauss J, Duncan Thomas et al. Quality of health care, survival and health outcomes in Ghana. *Journal of Health Economics* 1996; 15: 333–357.

concluded that African children in communities with more doctors tended to be taller .

– The socio-professional characteristics of doctors

45 volunteer nephrologists from ten African countries across five regions participated in this study (figure 13):

- **North Africa:** 55.56 % (Morocco 24.4 %, Tunisia 22.2 %, Egypt: 8.9 %)
- **West Africa:** 15.56 % (Mauritania 6.7 %, Senegal 8.9 %)
- **East Africa:** 4.44 % (Burundi 4.44 %)
- **Central Africa:** 17.78 % (Chad 4.4 %, Cameroon 8.9 %, Gabon 4.4 %)
- **Southern Africa:** 6.67 % (Mozambique 6.67 %)

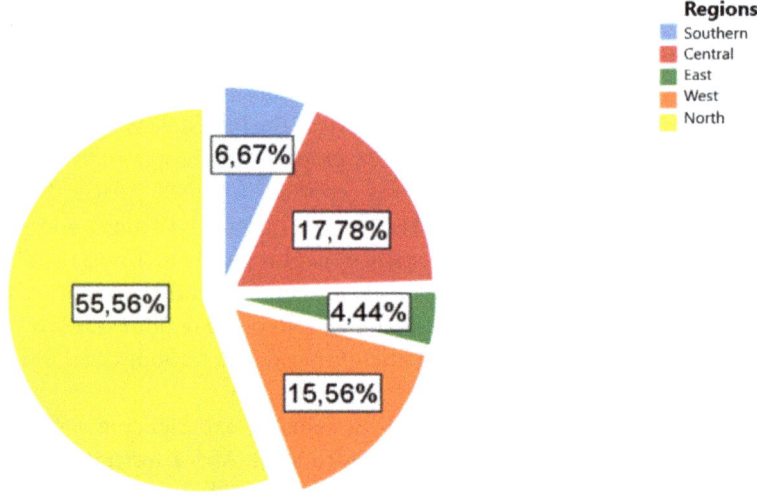

Figure 13: The distribution of doctors across African regions

– Age and seniority in professional practice:

The completion of our study was made possible by the enthusiasm and collaboration of a group of young African nephrologists. They saw our survey as an opportunity to have their voices heard and to bring attention to the obstacles they face in their profession.

The average age of the participating nephrologists was 38.84 ± 7.65 years, and their ages ranged from 26 to 58 years. The largest age group was between 30 and

40 years, making up 46.7 % of doctors. On average, these doctors had 9.30 ± 5.83 years of service, ranging from 2 to 27 years. In addition, 43.2 % of them had been in service for 5 to 10 years.

It is important to note that younger healthcare practitioners showed more interest in participating in studies that evaluated their hospitals or healthcare systems, as observed in several publications. For instance, a study examining the perceptions of Indian doctors and managers regarding hospital social responsibility found that 33.9 % of the respondents with less than 5 years of work experience were the most represented category. Similarly, another study conducted in Iran on the perceptions of CSR in hospitals found that the average age of the participants (doctors and administrators) willing to be interviewed was 34.5 years.

However, little is known about the age distribution of nephrologists in Africa. In the United States, the 40–44 years age group is the largest age cohort for nephrologists, followed by the 35–39 age group[347].

– Gender

On the whole, there is a global increase in the number of women enrolling in medical schools and the percentage of female nephrologists. In our study, 53.49 % of the participating nephrologists were men and 46.51 % were women, resulting in a male/female ratio of 1.15. Gabon and Morocco stood out as the countries with the highest percentage of female participating nephrologists, with 100 % and 70 % respectively.

A report by the American Society of Nephrology[348] highlighted the increasing representation of women in the field of nephrology. Although historically the percentage of women in nephrology was lower, there has been a notable rise in the number of female trainee nephrologists since 2012, due to the increasing number of female graduates from medical schools. However, the report also indicated that nephrology is still male-dominated.

Additionally, surveys assessing doctors' perceptions of hospital corporate social responsibility revealed that the majority of respondents were male. Indeed, research in the Western world has shown that gender influences doctors' involvement in surveys and their responses to

---

347 Salsberg E, Masselink L, Wu X. *The US nephrology workforce: developments and trends*. Washington, DC: American Society of Nephrology; 2014.
348 Eleanor Lederer. Women in nephrology today. *Clinical Journal of the American Society of Nephrology* 2018; 13: 1755–1756.

questionnaires[349,350,351]. The findings varied depending on the likelihood of receiving payment for participating in the study. However, data from research in developed countries indicates that female doctors were more likely to participate in surveys and polls. The dominance of male participants in our study could be attributed to the lower number of women in the field of nephrology, especially in Africa.

– The practice sector and major activities

As with patients, we chose hospitals based on our survey framework, focussing on state-run regional and university hospitals. The objective was to evaluate their social responsibility, and more specifically their professional responsibility. This explains why nephrologists affiliated with these hospitals were included in our study. Thus, 61.9 % of the surveyed doctors were from regional public hospitals while 38.1 % were from university hospitals.

The university nephrologists participating in the study were from Morocco, Egypt, Tunisia, and Chad. 38.64 % of them reported that their work combined clinical nephrology and hemodialysis in equal proportions. 20.45 % were exclusively devoted only to dialysis, 22.73 % were focussed on clinical nephrology, and 18.18 % were involved in both kidney transplantation and clinical nephrology.

36.4 % of the participating nephrologists from Morocco and 50 % from Senegal stated that their major work area was dialysis; 100 % from Egypt and 40 % from Tunisia stated that kidney transplantation and nephrology were their major work areas. The majority of other nephrologists practiced nephrology and dialysis in equal proportions.

The doctors included in our study did not practise peritoneal dialysis or focus solely on kidney transplantation. Generally, the practice of these activities remains limited across the African continent. The range of activities performed by the nephrologists participating in this study reveals some of the challenges associated with kidney replacement therapy. Kidney transplantation in Africa is hindered by many obstacles, such as the limited availability of specialised doctors

---

349 Cunningham CT, Quan H, Hemmelgarn B et al. Exploring physician specialist response rates to web-based surveys. *BMC Medical Research Methodology* 2015; 15: 32.
350 Delnevo CD, Abatemarco DJ, Steinberg MB. Physician response rates to a mail survey by specialty and timing of incentive. *American Journal of Preventive Medicine* 2004; 26(3): 234–236.
351 Fan W, Yen Z. Factors affecting response rates of the web survey: A systematic review. *Computers in Human Behavior* 2009; 26(2): 132–139.

and surgeons, distrust in the healthcare system, and high costs. For instance, the financial burden of transplantation and post-operative care, including anti-rejection immunosuppressive therapy, on kidney patients in Africa overshadows the benefits of transplantation over dialysis, which is commonly observed in high-income countries.

In several African countries, healthcare professionals are urging their governments to advance transplantation programmes. Some of these countries are currently developing this therapeutic solution, which emphasises the importance of respecting societal values by safeguarding the well-being of donors and recipients. Moreover, this initiative not only helps to improve the healthcare system and ensure universal health coverage but also strengthens the connection between the healthcare system and the public.

In comparison to other parts of the world, especially high-income countries, the costs of dialysis and transplantation in Africa are often higher in proportion to personal income or per capita health expenditure. For example, peritoneal dialysis (PD) is theoretically a cost-effective alternative for healthcare systems compared to hemodialysis. It can be performed at home without the need for machinery or electricity, making it an ideal choice in low-resource settings. However, PD is not a priority in Africa because it is more expensive and less profitable. This is due to the high cost of imported consumables, as well as the imposition of import duties and unofficial taxes, all of which are passed on to the consumer. Consequently, this technique is not widely adopted in Africa. While some countries use PD for short-term treatment of acute kidney failure, the high costs make long-term PD treatment nearly impossible to envision [352].

- Hospital size

The participating doctors were affiliated with hospitals of different sizes: 15.6 % were large-sized, 73.3 % were medium-sized, and 11.1 % were small-sized. Except for Mozambique, where most participants came from large hospitals, and Burundi, where most participants came from small hospitals, most doctors in the other countries came from medium-sized hospitals. This distribution reflects the common practice of nephrology in secondary (regional) and tertiary (university) healthcare facilities, which are typically of medium to large size.

- The doctors' perceptions of hospital social responsibility

---

352   Callegari J,·Antwi SB. Peritoneal dialysis as a mode of treatment for acute kidney injury in sub-Saharan Africa. *Blood Purification* 2013; 36: 226–230.

Analysing doctors' perceptions of hospital social responsibility is important for improving the quality of care and people's health. The findings indicate that the factors leading to the dissatisfaction of doctors could signal deeper quality issues in the healthcare system. In the field of nephrology, there has been limited rigorous research evaluating the nephrologists' perspectives on their practice or examining methods to enhance the quality of care. The evaluation of healthcare system performance often fails to consider the professionals' views of their work environment or the overall healthcare system quality[353,354]. The quality of services, including the impact of the work environment, is generally assessed in high and middle-income countries where the quality of services is well-established. In contrast, low- and lower-middle-income countries are facing different challenges, usually related to equal access to healthcare rather than to the quality of healthcare. Likewise, we examined the perceptions of nephrologists regarding the social responsibility of their hospitals in terms of professional obligations. We first evaluated their satisfaction with the quality of care , access to care, and the professional ethics of their hospitals.

*Quality of care:

The first aspect we looked at was how the participants perceived the quality of care. We examined the following three areas: the therapeutic management of patients, the hospital environment, and the care process.

- *The doctors' satisfaction with the outcomes of the therapeutic management of patients:* The provision of quality healthcare depends on having a sufficient number of skilled, dedicated, and motivated health professionals working in a well-resourced system. The WHO states that an effective healthcare system includes all organisations, individuals, and actions whose primary goal is to promote, restore, and maintain good health[355,356].

---

353 Ortiz-Prado E, Fors M, Henriquez-Trujillo. AR et al. Attitudes and perceptions of medical doctors towards the local health system: a questionnaire survey in Ecuador. *BMC Health Services Research* 2019; 19: 363.
354 Rotenstein LS, Huckman RS, Wagle NW. Making patients and doctors happier – the potential of patient-reported outcomes. *The New England Journal of Medicine* 2017; 377: 1309–1312.
355 Global strategy on human resources for health: workforce 2030. WHO; 2016.
356 Durán A, Kutzin J, Martin-Moreno JM et al. Understanding health systems: scope, functions and objectives. In: Health Syst Health Wealth Soc Well- NY Open Univ. Press. McGraw Hill; 2011, pp. 19–37.

A study conducted in India[357] found that the main motivator for doctors in their workplace is professional excellence. This finding aligns with Maslow's hierarchy of needs, indicating that once medical professionals have met their basic needs and established themselves in society, they can achieve self-actualisation through reaching higher levels of professional excellence. This was supported by a study[358] sponsored by the American Medical Association (AMA), which also found that delivering high quality healthcare is the main source of doctors' professional satisfaction. Overcoming barriers to quality care would benefit both patients and caregivers.

Furthermore, according to a study conducted by Parker and colleagues in the United States, nephrologists perceived nephrology as a challenging medical specialty with heavy patient care and limited clinician satisfaction[359].

- *The doctors' satisfaction with the hospital environment:* Healthcare systems depend on health professionals to provide healthcare services and establish an operational framework. Therefore, it is crucial to consider their views on their working environment, overall working conditions, public policies governing their work, and the flaws within their healthcare system.

In our study, we found that 53.3 % of doctors were dissatisfied with their hospital environment. Specifically, 15.6 % were very dissatisfied, 17.8 % were neutral, and only 13.3 % were satisfied. Except for Egyptian doctors who were neutral or satisfied in equal proportions, most nephrologists from the other surveyed countries were dissatisfied with the hospital environment.

Health professionals in many parts of the world are facing various challenges when delivering services. These include poor or inadequate infrastructure, limitations in their profession practice and overcrowded health departments with ever-increasing queues. While these problems may differ from country to country, most healthcare systems experience some degree of administrative and

---

357 Nirupam M. Attitudes and perceptions of medical doctors towards their jobs in the state of J&K, India. *International Journal of Health* 2007; 1(2).
358 Friedberg MW, Chen PG, Van Busum KR et al. factors affecting physician professional satisfaction and their implications for patient care, health systems, and health policy. *Rand Health Quarterly* 2014; 3(4): 1.
359 Parker MG, Pivert KA, Ibrahim T. Molitoris recruiting the next generation of nephrologists. *Advances in Chronic Kidney Disease* 2013 July; 20(4): 326–335.

organisational issues, regardless of the income level or standard of living of citizens[360,361,362]

The shortage of skilled health workers, equipment, and modern infrastructure is one of the main challenges in African healthcare systems[363]. Most hospitals, especially in the sub-Saharan part of the continent, have underdeveloped infrastructure and still rely on traditional, often inefficient equipment. This is a major contributing factor to doctors' dissatisfaction with the work environment and general condition of health facilities, as noted in our survey.

- *The doctors' satisfaction with the care process*: Our study revealed that 37.8 % of doctors were satisfied with the care process in their hospitals, 15.6 % were neutral, 35.6 % were dissatisfied, and 11.1 % were very dissatisfied. The majority of doctors from Egypt, Senegal, and Tunisia were satisfied with care delivery, while those from Burundi and Mauritania were generally dissatisfied. Nephrologists from other countries provided mixed responses.

Several authors pointed out that the quality of the care process has an impact on both doctors and patients in resource-limited countries. The provision of care in these countries is often hindered by shortages of staff and logistics such as medical analysis laboratories, patient management protocols, staff training, and supervision. These challenges, combined with the high number of patients, make it difficult for doctors to always provide optimal.

A satisfactory care process involves providing care in line with current scientific knowledge and the standards set by the learned societies, without any delays that could compromise treatment protocols. Delays may be caused by medication shortages, lack of necessary tests for diagnosis or follow-up, and non-availability of hospital beds.

---

360   Ortiz-Prado E, Fors M, Henriquez-Trujillo. AR et al. Attitudes and perceptions of medical doctors towards the local health system: a questionnaire survey in Ecuador. *BMC Health Services Research* 2019; 19: 363.
361   Squires D, Anderson C. US health care from a global perspective: spending, use of services, prices, and health in 13 countries. Commonwealth Fund 2015; 15: 1–16.
362   Guttmann A, Schull MJ, Vermeulen MJ et al. Association between waiting times and short term mortality and hospital admission after departure from emergency department: population based cohort study from Ontario, Canada. *BMJ* 2011; 342: d2983.
363   Poor health systems and lack of infrastructure paralyses health care in Africa. AFRIC Editorial; Dec. 2018. Available at: <https://afric.online/5626-poor-health-systems-and-lack-of-infrastructure-paralyses-health-care-in-africa/>.

In an Asian study,[364] it was found that doctor dissatisfaction with the care process was mainly due to difficulties in adhering to recommended treatment protocols and the lack of logistical support. In Africa, doctors report a lack of medicines, patient poverty, and an inability to perform the necessary laboratory tests required for treatment protocols. Most of these tests are either non-available or expensive as they are often performed in private laboratories or subcontracted abroad. Moreover, the large number of patients means difficulties securing hospital beds, leading to more delays in the therapeutic management[365].

- The nephrologists' responses to open-ended questions about the "Quality of Care"

"I am only satisfied with the care outcome of my patients when it is adequately provided according to the rules of good practice and when the treatment protocols are well-conducted, which is not always the case."

"No, I'm not always satisfied with the therapeutic management of patients because it very often meets obstacles that disrupt the continuity of care. Many kidney diseases require long-term treatment, and there is often a lack of medication adherence, leading to treatment interruptions and to patients being lost to follow-up, which is really frustrating!"

"In our department, we do our best, and despite our limited resources, we still manage to save lives and achieve good results. So, I can say that our medical care is quite satisfactory although we would like to improvements and work in better conditions."

"The general conditions in the hospital make it difficult to provide proper patient care. The departments are small and poorly equipped, with malfunctioning ultrasounds and scanners. There is a lack of anatomopathologists, hematologists, and cardiovascular surgeons on site. There are times when the hospital exceeds its capacity for patient rooms, leading to hygiene and organisational issues."

"No one can deny that the hospital is offering little comfort to patients. We are working to remedy this by reducing the length of hospital stays, although it's challenging. The care process is getting disrupted by the lack of medical tests in the hospital laboratory and by the financial constraints of patients who are unable to afford to them in external (private) laboratories. This leads to unnecessary long hospital stays and make conditions more difficult for patients."

---

364 Islam F, Rahman A, Halim A et al. Perceptions of health care providers and patients on quality of care in maternal and neonatal health in fourteen Bangladesh government healthcare facilities: a mixed-method study. *BMC Health Services Research* 2015; 15: 237.

365 Chodzaza E, Bultemeier K. Service providers' perception of the quality of emergency obsteric care provided and factors identified which affect the provision of quality care. *Malawi Medical Journal* 2010; 22(4): 104–111.

"In addition to logistical and financial concerns, the care process would be much easier if we interacted more with patients, and if we informed and convinced them about the proposed treatment protocols. This becomes hard when dealing with a large number of patients and facing language and dialect barriers..."

*Access to healthcare:

Access to healthcare is a major problem in developing countries, especially for low-income people who often struggle to obtain health services[366].

Care accessibility was the second dimension examined in our study. It was assessed by investigating doctors' satisfaction with three key factors: their patients' waiting times for consultations or hospital admissions, the cost of care (including treatments, biological and radiological tests, among others), and the availability of necessary treatment at the hospital.

- *The doctors' satisfaction with waiting times / referral times:* In our study, only 33.3 % of doctors expressed satisfaction with the waiting times or referral times of their patients to receive consultation or hospitalisation in their health facility. 15.6 % were neutral about these delays, 24.4 % were dissatisfied, and 26.7 % were very dissatisfied. The majority of nephrologists from Egypt were satisfied with their patients' waiting times. In contrast, nephrologists from Burundi and Mozambique reported dissatisfaction. Nephrologists from other countries gave mixed responses.

The doctors' satisfaction with patients' waiting times varies significantly between countries. According to a recent study conducted in Saudi Arabia, the majority of nephrologists believed that patients arrived on time and were satisfied with the referral time from primary care facilities to hospitals with specialised nephrology services.

However, studies[367] conducted in many developed countries such as Canada, United States, the United Kingdom, and Australia consistently show longer waiting times, especially in emergency departments due to the high number of patients. These longer waits can lead to delays in managing serious conditions

---

366   Peters DH, Garg A, Bloom G et al. Poverty and access to health care in developing countries. *Annals of the New York Academy of Sciences* 2008; 1136(1): 161–171.
367   Guttmann A, Schull MJ, Vermeulen MJ et al. Association between waiting times and short term mortality and hospital admission after departure from emergency department: population based cohort study from Ontario, Canada. *BMJ* 2011; 342: d2983.

that usually require hospitalisation. Frustrated by long waits, up to 10 % of patients leave without seeing a doctor, receiving a diagnosis or getting treatment, which can have serious consequences. Thus, prolonged stays in the emergency department reflect the increased waiting times for consultation or hospitalisation in developed countries. Additionally, the risk of death rises with each extra hour of waiting, especially for elderly patients. Analyses also indicate that reducing the average waiting time by one hour could have potentially saved the lives of 6.5 % of patients with severe conditions.

Late presentation and referral of patients with chronic kidney disease (CKD) to nephrologists pose significant barriers to accessing nephrology care. With estimated prevalence between 30 % and 82 % worldwide, late presentation and referral are on the rise, despite the well-known benefits of early nephrology care[368]. The time from initial consultation to starting dialysis varies from 3 to 12 months. Notably, the highest prevalence is observed in developing countries, particularly in sub-Saharan Africa. For instance, in Douala, Cameroon, , 3 out of every 4 CKD patients present late for nephrology care. Consequently, up to 96 % of late-referred patients require emergency dialysis on a temporary catheter, leading to higher hospitalisation rates and a poor short-term survival rate.

The quality of the healthcare system, the density of nephrologists in a specific area, and proximity to nephrology centres are important factors that impact patient referral and presentation.

However, studies conducted in Africa[369,370,371] revealed that late referrals were due to a number of factors. 64.15 % of cases were attributed to general doctors failing to screen for kidney impairment and 35.85 % were due to failure to refer patients at an early stage of the disease. Additionally, 81.25 % of patients were responsible for late presentation by not seeking hospital care, and 18.75 % of

---

368 Halle MP, Nyongbella J, Fouda H et al. Factors associated with late presentation of patients with chronic kidney disease in nephrology consultation in Cameroon-a descriptive cross-sectional study. *Renal Failure* 2019; 41(1): 384–392.

369 Halle MP, Nyongbella J, Fouda H et al. Factors associated with late presentation of patients with chronic kidney disease in nephrology consultation in Cameroon-a descriptive cross-sectional study. *Renal Failure* 2019; 41(1): 384–392.

370 Naicker S. End-stage renal disease in sub-Saharan Africa. *Ethnicity & Disease* 2009;19:S1–13–5.

371 Halle MPE, Kengne AP, Ashuntantang G. Referral of patients with kidney impairment for specialist care in a developing country of sub-Saharan Africa. *Renal Failure* 2009; 31: 341–348.

patients did not respect the decision of transfer to a specialised nephrology centre.

It is important to consider the socio-cultural context, as in African societies, the disease is often associated with certain factors such as the presence of symptoms, a lack of understanding of the silent nature of kidney disease, high economic constraints (including individual spending on medical costs and the low rate of health coverage), low levels of education, and a preference for comparatively cheaper traditional medicine. These factors may justify the high rates of non-recourse to hospitals for treatment. On the other hand, late referral to nephrology consultation might be explained by denial of the disease and limited knowledge about the dialysis process, which can cause fear and a rejection of the technique, as highlighted by a number of authors.

- *The doctors' satisfaction with the cost of care*: 24.4 % of doctors in our study were satisfied with the cost of care at their hospitals, 37.8 % were neutral, 20 % were dissatisfied, and 13.3 % were very dissatisfied. Except for Egypt, Mauritania, and Senegal, where doctors were mostly satisfied with the cost of treatment, the rest were either neutral (Morocco, Mozambique, and Tunisia) or dissatisfied (Burundi, Cameroon, and Chad).

The low satisfaction rates of nephrologists with the cost of care in Africa are understandable, given that such care is unaffordable to patients and hinders disease management.

In developing countries, despite investments in public health, out-of-pocket expenditure continues to make up a significant part of total healthcare expenditure. In Ecuador, for example, out-of-pocket expenditure on health accounts for an average of 7.2 % of total family income. Wealthier families spend more on private consultations and insurance, which makes up 71 % of health expenditure. Conversely, poorer families spend more out-of-pocket for medicines than wealthier families, indicating lesser access to health coverage and medical care, and explaining the widespread self-medication in these communities.[372] Thus, quality care at lower cost is becoming a necessity all over the world, particularly in resource-limited countries.

Hospitals are social organisations with an economic dimension, rather than economic organisations with a social dimension. Improving the efficiency and

---

372 Ortiz-Prado E, Fors M, Henriquez-Trujillo. AR et al. Attitudes and perceptions of medical doctors towards the local health system: a questionnaire survey in Ecuador. *BMC Health Services Research* 2019; 19: 363.

organisation of healthcare services is the most significant contribution hospital managers can make, ensuring better access and affordability of care for all segments of society. Healthcare system decision-makers and hospital managers have a moral obligation to work on increasing access to care and introducing new measures to curb pharmaceutical expenditure without compromising the quality of care.

Cameron et al.[373] estimate that 89 % of the cost of medicines could be saved in developing countries by using lowest-priced generic equivalents. Strategies to promote generic prescribing and delivery in France led to estimated annual savings of 1 billion € in 2007, 0.905 billion € in 2008, and 1.01 billion € in 2009. In addition, this had a positive impact on medication adherence, significantly affecting disease progression and overall population health[374,375].

Studies in Nigeria[376] showed a low rate of generic prescribing despite underfunding in the healthcare sector. Out-of-pocket expenditure is the main form of health expenditure among the population, accounting for up to 62 % of total health expenditure. These findings can be extrapolated to several African countries, explaining that policy makers' decisions and choices impact available medicines and on potential medication adherence, especially among patients with chronic diseases.

- *The doctors' satisfaction with the availability of treatment in the hospital*: 35.7 % of doctors were dissatisfied with the lack of essential treatment in their hospitals, and 23.8 % were very dissatisfied. Except for Egypt, where most of the surveyed doctors stated that treatment was available and free in their hospitals, and Morocco, where they were neutral about this issue, most nephrologists from the other countries were dissatisfied.

---

373 Cameron A, Mantel-Teeuwisse AK, Leufkens HG. Switching from originator brand medicines to generic equivalents in selected developing countries: how much could be saved? *Value in Health. The Journal of the International Society for Pharmacoeconomics and Outcomes Research* 2012; 15(5): 664–673.

374 Godman B, Abuelkhair M, Vitry A et al. Payers endorse generics to enhance prescribing efficiency; impact and future implications, a case history approach. *GaBI* 2012; 1(2): 21–35.

375 Briesacher BA, Andrade SE, Fouayzi H et al. Medication adherence and use of generic drug therapies. *The American Journal of Managed Care* 2009; 15(7): 450–456.

376 Fadare JO, Adeoti AO, Desalu OO et al. The prescribing of generic medicines in Nigeria: knowledge, perceptions and attitudes of physicians. *Expert Review of Pharmacoeconomics & Outcomes Research* 2016; 16(5): 639–650.

The dissatisfaction of doctors with the availability of treatment is common in developing countries. In a South American study, 53.5 % of the surveyed doctors complained about limited resources in public hospitals. Moreover, 71.8 % of the respondents mentioned shortcomings in the national essential medicines list, particularly with regard to the availability of some medicines such as anticancer drugs, antibiotics, and antihypertensives. Additionally, 57.5 % expressed concerns about the quality of generic medicines available for treatment.

In Africa, the lack of medicines is due to weak and under-resourced healthcare systems, attributed to challenges of leadership, governance, and financing. Rampant corruption in medical products and technologies procurement systems, unreliable supply, unaffordable prices, irrational use, and wide variance in quality have contributed to the current situation, where 50 % of the population in the African region lacks access to essential medicines[377].

Furthermore, health financing in the region is characterised by low investment, lack of comprehensive, strategic health financing policies and plans, high direct out-of-pocket payments, lack of social security for the poor, weak financial management, inefficient use of resources, and weak coordination mechanisms.

- The nephrologists' responses to open-ended questions about the "Accessibility of Care"

> *"Waiting times in our hospital are not long, but we face issues with delayed consultations and referrals for patients. On the one hand, many patients don't show up in time for a number of reasons; on the other hand, health professionals fail to detect kidney disease early, leading to late management of the patient who is often seen at the stage of complications."*
>
> *"Waiting times are a problem here. As our facility serves a large part of the country, there is therefore a high demand for our services, resulting in full hospital beds, and extended waiting times for several days or weeks for specialised nephrology care."*
>
> *"I work in a small dialysis unit. Access to nephrology care is very complicated, as there is no nephrology department in the whole country."*
>
> *"Many patients don't show up early for consultation; they visit traditional healers first; hospital is their last resort."*
>
> *"There aren't enough nephrologists to meet the needs of all the people we serve, be it in terms of specialised consultations or hospitalisations. That's why waiting times are inevitably long."*

---

377   Kirigia JM, Barry SP. Health challenges in Africa and the way forward. *International Archives of Medicine* 2008; 1: 27.

"The cost of care far exceeds the household budget. Since most patients don't have health insurance, they are forced to pay the hospital bill. They often leave treatment incomplete despite medical advice due to the lack of resources. That is not easy."
"The aid scheme for the most deprived in our country has made a lot of things easier. Patients have access to almost all services in the hospital, such as dialysis, but not anti-rejection treatment following the transplant. So, I would say that the situation is improving. It is definitely better than before."
"Many medical check-ups and treatments are lacking in the hospital. I think that it's the same for all specialties."
"Antibiotics, painkillers and antihypertensives aren't always available. It's frustrating because these are basic and essential medicines."

*Professional ethics:

– *Measures to protect patient privacy*: Medical confidentiality is a crucial aspect of ethical professional practice. Our study found that 40 % of doctors were satisfied with the measures in place to protect patient privacy, while 35.6 % were neutral, 20 % were dissatisfied, and 4.4 % were very dissatisfied.

Most of the Senegalese doctors participating in the study were not satisfied with the hospital's efforts to respect patient privacy. Moroccan and Tunisian nephrologists, on the other hand, were mostly neutral. When responding to the open-ended questions in the study, many African nephrologists reported several shortcomings, including the poor quality of record management, little interest in the value of confidentiality, limited awareness among stakeholders, concerns about the impact of new technologies on patient privacy, and the dilemma of publishing scientific information without patients' informed consent.

While medical publications are crucial for sharing information among doctors, and for continuing medical education, ensuring privacy and restricting access to personal patient data are pressing concerns[378]. A recent paper by Philip Rosoff[379] discussed the challenges doctors face in respecting patient confidentiality while communicating relevant details of their cases. He raised the question of whether "the educational and scientific value of (some) case reports justifies the potential threat to personal privacy inherent in the format". This is particularly relevant because some case reports could inadvertently reveal the identities of patients,

---

378 Nylenna M, Riis P. Identification of patients in medical publications: need for informed consent. *British Medical Journal* 1991; 302: 1182.
379 Rosoff PM. Can the case report withstand ethical scrutiny? Hastings Center Report 2019; 49(6): 17–21.

especially those with a unique or chronic medical condition requiring frequent access to healthcare facilities. Such disclosure can have severe consequences for these individuals, including stigmatisation and social exclusion.

In medical journals, authors are required to obtain informed consent from patients before publishing their cases. These cases must be sufficiently interesting and important, and are subject subject to preliminary internal review by an institutional committee to ensure their significance and respect for confidentiality. If the paper fails to pass this stage, it does not proceed further. If it does pass, possibly with required confidentiality revisions, the draft will then be shared with the patient or their family for consent or decline for publication. If consent is given, the paper can be published. This procedure is crucial for avoiding potential consequences of breaching patient privacy[380,381].

On the other hand, medical records management plays a vital role in patient privacy. According to Mpho Ngoepe[382], medical records management is one of the key components of the quality and credibility of hospital care. Health professionals in Africa have expressed their dissatisfaction with the weak, slow, and inadequate hospital records management system. Evidence from Ethiopia[383] revealed that practitioners were dissatisfied with the quality of their hospital's records management system and its impact on the care process and data security.

A South African study[384] noted that despite all precautions, doctors were unsure of the security of records storage locations in hospitals. Patient folders were occasionally left unattended in consultation rooms, not archived in time, or misfiled. These incidents were attributed to the manual records management system and staff inattention. It was suggested to implement a more efficient

---

380   Nylenna M, Riis P. Identification of patients in medical publications: Need for informed consent. *British Medical Journal* 1991; 302: 1182.
381   Rosoff PM. Can the case report withstand ethical scrutiny? Hastings Center Report 2019; 49(6): 17–21.
382   Ngoepe M. An exploration of records management trends in the South African public sector. *Mousaion* 2009; 27: 116–136.
383   Wong REX, Bradley EH. Developing patient registration and medical records management system in Ethiopia. International journal for quality in health care 2009; 21(4): 253–258.
384   Mathebeni-Bokwe P. Management of medical records for healthcare service delivery at the Victoria Public Hospital in the Eastern Cape Province: South Africa (thesis). Alice (South Africa): Fort Hare univ.; 2015. Available at: <https://pdfs.semanticscholar.org/e888/2023a43f5266449c6eed35f092f02e47163f.pdf>.

electronic archiving system and raise professionals' awareness of patient confidentiality.

African authors[385] are warning of privacy risks posed by technological advances such as computerised filing, archiving, and telemedicine unless precautionary measures and ethical practices are adopted. For instance, computer storage of identifiable patient information may result in confidential patient data being accessed by commercial industries or the mass media. While technologies provide patient benefits, they also carry the potential for harm. Therefore, hospitals need to address new ethical challenges related to protecting patient confidentiality.

- *The doctors' perceptions of equity in healthcare delivery*: 17.8 % of doctors felt that patients were always treated fairly in hospitals, 44.4 % said that this was only occasional, and 6.7 % said that this was rarely the case. Most nephrologists from Burundi, Morocco, Mauritania, and Mozambique felt that patient care in their hospitals was only 'sometimes' fair. Most Tunisian and Senegalese nephrologists thought that their health facilities were generally fair. Most Egyptian doctors felt that their facilities were always fair in providing healthcare.

Equity in health in this context implies equitably providing specialised nephrological care, including costly kidney replacement therapy (dialysis and renal transplantation), in a resource-limited region where a significant part of healthcare costs fall on households. An equitable implementation of dialysis programmes should address issues of availability and acceptability. The main structural factors that affect equity of access to dialysis in different countries are the organisation of healthcare systems, overall health care spending, funding and delivery models of kidney replacement therapy (KRT), namely transplantation, hemodialysis, or peritoneal dialysis. An international group of experts[386] who studied equity of access to healthcare for end-stage kidney disease in Africa noted that equitable implementation of a health programmes such as KRT requires consideration of three elements: availability, affordability, and acceptability. The decision to implement such a programme is driven by the needs from the

---

385   Knapp van Bogaert D. Ethics CPD supplement: ethics in health care: confidentiality and information technologies. *South African Family Practice* 2014; 56(1) (Suppl 1): S3–S5.
386   Van Biesen W, Jha V, Abu-Alfa AK. Considerations on equity in management of end-stage kidney disease in low- and middle-income countries. *Kidney International Supplements* 2020; 10: e63–e71.

public in relation to the local context to ensure equitable service delivery for all patients[387].

There are global inequities in the provision of KRT, leading to differences in the prevalence of treated end-stage kidney disease (ESKD) across regions. The funding and organisation of healthcare systems greatly impact equitable access to renal care. Low- and middle-income countries often lack the financial, logistic, and labour force capacity to provide such care at scale. Additionally, the availability of these treatments does not guarantee accessibility, which is driven by personal, family, geographical, and societal factors. In low-income countries, there is a typically minimal involvement of the public sector[388,389]. Market dynamics govern access to kidney disease therapy and result in a high incidence of out-of-pocket expenditure. Conversely, in high-income countries, kidney disease therapy is predominantly funded by the public sector.

There is a strong correlation between a country's gross domestic product (GDP) and the prevalence of treated kidney disease. However, differences in the implementation of health policies also affect care delivery regardless of the country's wealth status. For instance, despite having similar incomes, South Africa's total healthcare expenditure (40 %) is significantly lower than in Thailand (75 %). The implementation of universal access to replacement therapy has succeeded in Thailand, while it is still restricted in South Africa[390].

Affordability is a major issue contributing to inequity in low- and middle-income countries. The WHO estimates that a minimal healthcare spending per person of 271 USD (range: 74–984 USD), or the allocation of 7.5 % (2.1 %–20.5 %) of GDP on healthcare is needed to achieve the health-related Sustainable Development Goals. Since GDP is not evenly distributed across the population,

---

387 Essue BM, Laba M, Knaul F et al. Economic burden of chronic ill health and injuries for households in low- and middle-income countries. In: Jamison DT, Gelband H, Horton S, et al., eds. *Disease control priorities: Improving health and reducing poverty*. 3rd ed. Washington, DC: The International Bank for Reconstruction and Development/ The World Bank; 2017.

388 Moosa MR, Kidd M. The dangers of rationing dialysis treatment: the dilemma facing a developing country. *Kidney International* 2006; 70: 1107–1114.

389 Garcia-Garcia G, Garcia-Bejarano H, Breien-Coronado H et al. End-stage renal disease in Mexico. In: Garcia-Garcia G, Agodoa L, Norris K, eds. *Chronic kidney disease in disadvantaged populations*. New York, NY: Elsevier; 2017: 77–82.

390 *Van Biesen W, Jha V, Abu-Alfa AK. Considerations on equity in management of end-stage kidney disease in low- and middle-income countries. Kidney Int. Suppl. 2020; 10: e63–e71.*

healthcare access inequities can persist even when an adequate average budget per capita is achieved.

It is estimated that about 188 million people in low- and middle-income countries experience catastrophic health expenses annually due to kidney diseases. The cost of replacement therapy per capita far exceeds the GDP, the minimal availability of dialysis, and the absence of sustainable funding models lead financial hardship for many families[391].

Furthermore, considering ethical and societal standards, the WHO emphasises that the basic needs of the population should met when implementing expensive healthcare technologies. Moreover, there is a debate among experts about whether kidney replacement therapy should be developed in regions with limited access to essential health services, as it could worsen overall health inequity. It should also be noted that failing to promote these therapies in public hospitals might encourage the private sector to step in and expand, especially at the level of dialysis. This could worsen inequity because certain patients will always be able to afford treatment, while the financially disadvantaged will end up in an even worse situation due to high out-of-pocket expenses.

- *The doctors' perceptions of care delivery regardless of patients' ability to pay:* In our survey, 15.6 % of doctors thought that hospitals always provided care regardless of patients' ability to pay, 6.7 % thought this was usually the case, 37.8 % thought it happened only occasionally, 22.2 % thought it was rare, and 17.8 % said it was never possible.

The majority of surveyed Egyptian doctors reported that care delivery in their hospitals was always fair. However, most doctors from Mozambique and Tunisia indicated that it was only "sometimes" observed, while those from Burundi stated that it was never observed in their hospitals.

Notably, the responses to open-ended questions on this topic were insightful. Most interviewed doctors expressed their commitment to providing care regardless of their patients' socio-economic status. Still, there is clear inequity gap between patients based on income level. Financially disadvantaged patients struggle to afford prescribed treatments, blood tests, and radiology tests. Additionally, low-income patients requiring dialysis face long waiting lists due to the inability to access private health facilities. There is also inequity in access

---

391 *Van Biesen W, Jha V, Abu-Alfa AK. Considerations on equity in management of end-stage kidney disease in low- and middle-income countries. Kidney Int. Suppl.* 2020; 10: e63–e71.

to kidney transplantation, as patients without health coverage cannot afford the necessary anti-rejection treatment, which they must take after transplantation and for the rest of their life. These findings support previous reports on the challenges African populations face in accessing healthcare .

When asked open-ended questions, many African nephrologists expressed discomfort with this topic, as follows:

> *"It's difficult to speak about respecting patient privacy when the records management system is outdated and deficient."*
>
> *"We take great care in sharing patient information and data, but I can't guarantee that the entire medical team – the nurses and ward staff – is doing the same thing."*
>
> *"We rarely discuss this matter within our team. My response is a personal one, so I can't comment on the hospital's compliance with patient confidentiality."*
>
> *"Our inventory locations and archiving systems aren't optimal. It's difficult to say that patient data is well-protected."*
>
> *"We do our best to protect patient information, but honestly, this matter isn't a top priority for the hospital. We seldom talk about it."*
>
> *"A computer system has been implemented to allow access to the patients' medical records from any department. So, access to this data has become much easier. However, I can't comment on confidentiality in this situation."*
>
> *"We published a case report without patient consent a couple of years ago. That was a long time ago. We weren't aware of that, and we had no ethics committee."*
>
> *"Do all publications involving patient data go through the ethics committee? No. I'm sure they don't. We try to respect confidentiality and research ethics as much as possible, but not all our publications have been approved by the committee."*

– The nephrologists' responses to open-ended questions about the "Equity of Care"

> *"We are doing our best to treat patients equitably, but we must face the reality that we can't conduct all the necessary check-ups and provide all treatments within hospital. Consequently, despite our best intentions, patients with more financial resources will have better access to care."*
>
> *"Equity isn't solely within our control. In fact, it's hard to talk about equity in such a context. As you and I well know, it isn't possible to prescribe a treatment that requires close-range biological tests to a patient living in a rural area far away from laboratories. Thus, because the first treatment is simply unmanageable, we often have to prescribe other less effective treatments. This can be extrapolated to many other clinical situations. Is this fair?*
>
> *"A patient with no health coverage and with few financial means can't aspire to ever be transplanted. He will end his life in dialysis, which is again a reality. He may be young and have parents or brothers and sisters willing to offer him a kidney, but it won't be possible unless he can afford the anti-rejection treatment for life. So, frankly, I don't think that such a situation is fair."*

"Here, in the dialysis department, we keep a waiting list, and prioritise poor patients based on the degree of urgency. The decision-making process for admitting a dialysis patient is transparent and fair."

"I don't think this issue is limited to the public hospital or to healthcare providers. Without a universal health coverage system, equitable healthcare delivery cannot be ensured. The poorest will always be treated unfairly in a way or another."

"Even if the patient manages to find a place for dialysis, there will still be monthly or quarterly medical check-ups to be done. He will often need treatment for anemia and other kidney failure complications. As you know, we are talking about expensive medicines not available in hospital for which patients pay out-of-pocket. And of course, treatment for those who can't afford it will be less adequate."

– The doctors' perceptions of hospital social responsibility

As our findings indicated, 60 % of practitioners believed that their hospitals were not socially responsible, 28.89 % saw that their hospitals' social responsibility was average, and only 8.89 % saw that it was good (figure 14).

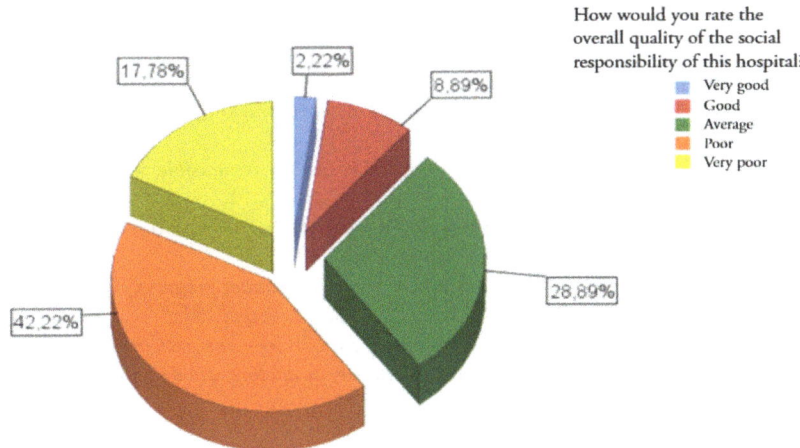

Figure 14: The doctors' perceptions of hospital social responsibility

According to the feedback from most Egyptian and Tunisian doctors, their hospitals' social responsibility was considered average, while Senegalese nephrologists rated it as good. Doctors from Gabon and Morocco had mixed opinions. Doctors from other countries generally felt that their hospitals were not socially responsible.

The averages scores of different items showed that doctors were generally dissatisfied with the three dimensions (quality, accessibility, and professional ethics) and with their hospitals' social responsibility.

In contrast, several other studies[392,393] considered the professional aspect of social responsibility as part of the core missions, requirements, or even basic obligations of hospitals. They also studied other aspects like leadership, marketing, external procedures, and the environment.

A study[394] exploring the perceptions of Iranian health professionals over their hospitals' social responsibility found that the hospitals' internal stakeholders were more interested in internal procedures, quality, care processes, and professional ethics. The study revealed a moderate level of satisfaction in these dimensions, but with a notable difference in perceptions. While managers believed that hospitals were adequately fulfilling their responsibilities, staff expected more efforts to improve the performance of their healthcare facilities. This was also highlighted by other authors[395].

- Nephrologists' responses to open-ended questions about their perceptions of hospital social responsibility

"I would say that the hospital where I work has average social responsibility in terms of professional obligations. There is much room for improvement in terms of workforce, materials, logistics, and organisation…"

"It wouldn't be truthful to say that our hospital is socially responsible; we are short of both financial means and strategy."

"With real determination and high-quality managers, our hospital could be socially responsible. Our biggest issue is a human resource problem."

"We are doing everything within our power. There is gradual progress. And while it requires patience, the hospital is becoming more socially responsible."

"Our hospital is socially responsible because we don't deny our patients the right to care; they have unrestricted access to it. While we, as doctors, are doing our best, the quality of care doesn't solely depend on us."

---

392 Abreu R, David F, Crowther D. Corporate social responsibility is urgently needed in health care. *Social Responsibility Journal* 2005; 1(3/4): 225–240.

393 Keyvanara M, Sajadi HS. Social responsibility of the hospitals in Isfahan city, Iran: results from a cross-sectional survey. *International Journal of Health Policy and Management* 2015; 4(8): 517–522.

394 Keyvanara M, Sajadi HS. Social responsibility of the hospitals in Isfahan city, Iran: Results from a cross-sectional survey. *International Journal of Health Policy and Management* 2015; 4(8): 517–522.

395 Bhuiyan A. Community health providers and their social responsibility. *International Journal of Gynecology & Obstetrics* 2009; 107: S128

"I must admit that I don't have a definitive answer to this question. There are limitations and flaws, but there are also significant efforts being made that shouldn't be disparaged. For an answer, I would say that the social responsibility of our hospital is average."

We investigated the correlation between doctors' perceptions of different dimensions of hospital social responsibility (quality, accessibility, and ethics) and their perceptions of hospital social responsibility using multilevel linear regression. This analysis revealed that only an item relative to the "accessibility" dimension (cost of treatment p: 0.039) showed a positive correlation. This means that a doctor could be satisfied with the quality or ethics of their hospital yet still judge the hospital as not socially responsible. However, an exception to this is the cost of care: a doctor who is satisfied with the cost of care at the hospital level is generally satisfied with the social responsibility of the hospital and vice versa. These results reveal the overall dissatisfaction of nephrologists with their hospitals, as indicated in several publications[396,397,398] about the perceptions of African doctors. The dissatisfaction is often attributed to the general working conditions in the hospital, the care process, and the Workload (table 9).

Table 9: Correlations between doctors' perceptions of hospital social responsibility and their satisfaction with its dimensions (multi-level linear regression models)

Coefficients[a]	Non-standardised coefficients		p
	A	Standard error	
Hospital	-,004	,423	,992
Gender	,103	,387	,793
Age (in years)	-,055	,051	,299
Job tenure (in years)	,055	,068	,428
Sector	,149	,398	,712

(fortgeführt)

---

396 Suliman AA, Eltom M, Elmadhoun WM. Factors affecting job satisfaction among junior doctors working at teaching hospitals in River Nile State, Sudan. *Journal of Public Health and Emergency* 2017; 1: 79.
397 Tadese T, Mohamed A, Mengistie A. Assessment of factors influencing job satisfaction among health care providers, federal police referral hospital, Addis Ababa, Ethiopia. *Ethiopian Journal of Health Development* 2015; 29: 119–126.
398 Amoran OE, Omokhodion FO, Dairo MD et al. Job satisfaction among primary health care workers in three selected local government areas in southwest Nigeria. Niger J Med 2005; 14: 195–199.

Table 9: Fortsetzung

Coefficients[a]			
Quality	,079	,272	,775
Satisfaction with the therapeutic management.	,087	,287	,765
Satisfaction with the hospital environment and conditions	,513	,349	,159
Satisfaction with the care process			
Accessibility	-,360	,200	,088
Satisfaction with the patients' waiting times	,619	,278	,039
Satisfaction with the costs of treatment	,029	,216	,896
Satisfaction with the availability of medicines in the hospital			
Ethics	-,065	,254	,801
Satisfaction with measures taken to protect patient privacy	,220	,284	,448
Satisfaction with equal access to healthcare	-,228	,318	,482
Satisfaction with access to healthcare regardless of ability to pay			
A. Dependent variable: Perception of hospital social responsibility			

– Correlations between doctors' attributes and their perceptions of hospital social responsibility

The statistical analysis of our findings showed no significant correlations between the doctors' socio-professional attributes and their perceptions of their hospitals' social responsibility.

A study conducted in India[399] found that doctors in the youngest age group tended to be more satisfied with their job and the hospital environment. This is likely because, at this stage of their careers, their primary focus is on achieving higher academic qualifications. However, satisfaction tended to decrease with more years of service (beyond 5 years), probably due to the changing dynamics of the medical work environment, causing a misalignment between personal goals and organisational priorities. On the other hand, it was observed that doctors working in teaching hospitals generally had a better perception of their hospitals'

---

399 Nirupam M. Attitudes and Perceptions of Medical Doctors Towards Their Jobs in the State of J&K, India International Journal of Health 2007; 1, No.2.

social responsibility. In addition, recent studies[400,401] clearly demonstrated that doctors' perceptions of the quality of healthcare facilities were influenced by their countries' economy, the level of the healthcare system, and the quality of its financing. However, these factors were not observed in our work.

- Correlations between countries' socio-economic data and doctors' perceptions of hospital social responsibility

The statistical analysis of these correlations indicated that there were no significant differences in the doctors' perceptions of hospital social responsibility based on the country's income (p: 0. 262, CI: 95 %), per capita health expenditure (PPP in US dollars) (p: 0.118, CI: 95 %), and per capita public expenditure on education (in % GDP) (p: 0.632, CI: 95 %).

- Comparison of patients' and nephrologists' perceptions of hospital social responsibility

This comparison revealed that the average scores were slightly better among patients than among doctors, with statistically significant differences for all items. Patients also had a more positive perception of the social responsibility of their hospitals compared to doctors. This difference was up to the limit of statistical significance (p:0.05). Despite feeling that their nephrologist provided adequate care, patients were often dissatisfied with the conditions and overall context of their healthcare. Similarly, doctors, while satisfied with the effects of their treatment, rarely had positive perceptions of hospital social responsibility.

When interpreting these results, it is important to consider the following points:

- Overall, patients were neutral in responding to several questions about the hospital environment and conditions, care process, availability and affordability of check-ups and treatments, waiting times, cost of treatment, equity of care, and professional ethics. However, they were generally satisfied with their nephrologist in terms of clinical examination, prescriptions, and treatment effects.

---

400 Solberg B, Tómasson K, Aasland O et al. Cross-national comparison of job satisfaction in doctors during economic recession. *Occupational Medicine* 2014; 64(8): 595–600.
401 Tyssen R, Palmer KS, Solberg IB. Physicians' perceptions of quality of care, professional autonomy, and job satisfaction in Canada, Norway, and the United States. *BMC Health Services Research* 2013; 13: 516.

- In contrast, doctors were more commonly dissatisfied with their hospital environment and conditions, availability and free delivery of medication, care process and waiting times.

As previously noted, some caution is necessary when interpreting the results. As reported by some authors[402,403,404], it is more likely that patients in good clinical condition, adhering to their doctors' instructions, participate more in attitude, perception and care satisfaction questionnaires, compared to dissatisfied patients. This may lead to a selection bias from the outset.

Furthermore, cultural factors and the level of education not only influence perceptions of the quality of care provided by the hospital but also affect patients' freedom of expression. Patients may fear the potential negative consequences of their responses, especially in a challenging context characterised by complicated access to healthcare. Additionally, kidney disease often requires frequent contact with the same care facility and caregivers over a long period of time, if not for life in the case of chronic dialysis. This could contribute to patients' caution or distrust in the survey, compared to doctors.

Most participating doctors were enthusiastic about taking part in our study and considered it an opportunity to highlight the difficulties hindering their work. They were also reassured by the measures we took to maintain their anonymity during data collection and analysis, which likely made them feel more comfortable expressing their dissatisfaction with several aspects.

---

402 Weaver M, Patrick DL, Markson LE et al. Issues in the measurement of satisfaction with treatment. *American Journal of Managed Care* 1997; 3: 579–594.
403 Morton RL, Tong A, Howard K et al. The views of patients and carers in treatment decision making for chronic kidney disease: systematic review and thematic synthesis of qualitative studies. *BMJ* 2010; 340: c112.
404 Morton RL, Tong A, Howard K et al. The views of patients and carers in treatment decision making for chronic kidney disease: systematic review and thematic synthesis of qualitative studies. *BMJ* 2010; 340: c112.

Chapter 4: The factors influencing hospital social responsibility

Nephrologists from seven countries, including Morocco, Tunisia, Mauritania, Gabon, Chad, Mozambique, and Burundi were asked open-ended questions about factors influencing hospital social responsibility, to which they provided in-depth answers. They saw that these factors were numerous, diverse, and varied as follows:

1. Patient-related factors

- **Socio-demographic factors**, particularly a patient's level of education and cultural background, have an impact on the care process from the perspective of doctors. These factors can lead to behaviours that hinder therapeutic management, such as turning to traditional medicine and herbalists, as well as struggling to understand therapeutic protocols. According to the interviewed doctors, these issues were more prevalent among patients with lower levels of education and could be attributed to the socio-cultural environment and the patients' beliefs.

    "Many patients don't understand what chronic disease is. They don't understand that it is not like a common illness such as bronchitis or sore throat for which they could visit the doctor once, get a perception, and then get better... With chronic kidney disease, long-term care is necessary; to maintain kidney function, regular appointments or even hospitalisation for complications are necessary. Kidney patients find this very difficult to manage, and feel frustrated about not being cured. What they want, instead, is to be cured. Hence, they often lose faith in the healthcare system quickly and turn to alternative healers whose treatments are more affordable. But this presents another issue."
    "It isn't always easy to explain the disease and treatment protocol to patients, especially if they are illiterate. It's always very difficult to convince them."
    "Enforcing dietary restrictions (such as a low-meat or low-potassium diet) is not easy. Moreover, despite our efforts and advice, and even if patients where I work listen to us, many keep using herbs and medicinal plants. It's the culture of this region, and won't change overnight."

- **Patient cooperation**: According to the interviewed doctors, a patient's adherence to caregivers' instructions regarding diet, medication, and appointment attendance are closely linked to their socio-demographic factors and significantly impacts the quality of care.

"Patients are not always very cooperative, which certainly complicates treatment. However, I think poor adherence isn't voluntary but rather a more or less direct consequence of the lack of resources. Once they can no longer afford treatment, they stop it, and unfortunately, this happens frequently!"

"To be honest, treatment adherence isn't very good here. I think that in addition to economic factors, doctors' instructions aren't always well understood. I have patients, for example, who stop their antihypertensive treatment as soon as there are no more tablets in the box. They need to be reminded regularly that this is a long-term medicine."

"Patients with chronic conditions get tired and do not always come for consultations. With time, they no longer take medicines correctly. You always have to check and re-explain…"

"I think if they had the financial means to pay for their treatment and enough education, their adherence to treatment would have been better…"

- **Kidney disease type**: Severe pathologies or those necessitating complex or long-term treatment protocols present a significant challenge for African doctors. Limited logistical and financial resources result in non-adherence among patients and their families.

"It's always more difficult to ensure patient adherence in the most serious illnesses requiring long-term treatment protocols and expensive medicines which are inconsistently available with frequent stock-outs…"

"It's not easy to convoke patients every fortnight or every month for new injections. Most patients live far away and may not have the possibility or the means to travel easily. So, they miss treatment appointments or are lost to follow-up very quickly. We often see them at advanced stages of the disease."

2. Doctor-related factors

- **Doctors' motivation and commitment**: Being motivated and committed is very crucial for the quality of care according to the interviewed doctors. The latter also expressed dissatisfaction with and demotivation by the conditions and environment of their hospitals.

"I like my job a lot, but I must admit that I'm not always motivated. The conditions in the hospital are difficult and really demotivating…"

"There aren't always enough places to receive patients; the medicines aren't always available; and the laboratory doesn't keep up. No, it's not always very motivating…"

"When I chose to become a doctor, I didn't think it would be this hard. To be honest, I don't have the same motivation as I did when I started."

- **Doctors' competence:** Respondents stressed the importance of foundational training, continuing medical education, and clinical experience to provide efficient and pertinent care. They expressed their dissatisfaction with the current medical education in universities, criticising its theoretical focus and reliance on outdated learning methods. In addition, they lamented the limited opportunities for continuing education, citing issues such as sparce access to international congresses, the absence of national congresses or training workshops in certain countries, and challenges in obtaining specialised scientific journals due to high membership fees.

    "In order to be successful, there are no secrets. You have to stay updated with the latest news in your field. How can you be so without access to specialised journals? I have access to a journal through my membership in the International Society of Nephrology, but I can't subscribe to two or three journals simultaneously. I can't afford it and there is a lack of institutional support."
    "In my workplace, there are hardly any scientific activities, congresses, medical events, round tables, or training workshops. Besides, we rarely receive invitations to international congresses. How can we keep ourselves informed about the latest scientific developments?"
    "The basic training at medical school was not very satisfactory. It mostly consisted of theoretical knowledge that didn't prepare us for real life patient care. I had to study nephrology abroad because it wasn't available here. Everything went well until I returned home. Things weren't easy in a completely different context. Neither the working conditions nor the diseases were the same!"
    "My basic training in nephrology had several gaps. I had to complete internships elsewhere and pursue additional inter-university degrees to fill those gaps."
    "There isn't a single book on nephrology in the medical school library, and it's generally very difficult to access such resources here."

- The lack of doctor training in effective communication and psychological management of patients with chronic diseases:

    "Communication is a pillar of the doctor-patient relationship. Many of us think that it should be integrated into the medical curriculum."
    "We need to have psychological knowledge and communication skills to manage our chronic patients. You need to have skills other than the technical and medical ones."

- **Absence of several specialties** such as vascular surgery, intensive care, laboratory service, pathological anatomy, and radiology among others.

> *"We can't do nephrology or dialysis without vascular surgeons, it's not possible. We send patients who have the means to neighbouring countries to have vascular access for dialysis. It's not that easy."*
>
> *"There are no vascular surgeons. This is certainly a big challenge for us. We also lack resuscitators. Can you imagine that? We manage as best we can when a patient needs intensive care unit treatment."*
>
> *"So many disciplines are missing, including surgeons, nutritionists, medical biologists, radiologists, and laboratory technicians."*

- Shortage of nephrologists and highly qualified nurses:

  > *"We are the only two nephrologists in the whole country, which should give you an idea of the present situation."*
  >
  > *"We are lacking nephrologists and nurses. You can well imagine that it can't be easy."*
  >
  > *"Our country has very few nephrologists. In recent years, we have recruited some Cuban nephrologists, but that has not solved the problem."*

- **Brain drain**, a significant problem in Africa, as particularly reported by sub-Saharan nephrologists.

  > *"There is a shortage of nephrologists in our regions, and those who are trained are being taken by the West!"*
  >
  > *"You can't expect to attract a nephrologist trained in Europe or the United States; these doctors hardly ever return. They have so many incentives there, making it hard for them to consider returning to their home country."*

3. Hospital-related factors

- **Leadership and governance**: The management and organisation of the hospital facility.

  > *"Nephrology at the hospital where I work isn't considered a priority specialty. When we communicate with decision-makers, we don't always feel that our voice is heard."*
  >
  > *"Our hospital managers don't help us at all."*
  >
  > *"We have got a director who is a good listener. That's a blessing. But he doesn't always have the means to help. It is very difficult to get machines repaired when they break down, as we don't have a maintenance contract. This complicates matters."*

- **Inadequate infrastructure,** insufficient number of specialised hospitals, non-availability, and non-local production of medicines and diagnostic tools.

"...The buildings are in a state of disrepair, and the departments are small and ill adapted for the large number of patients we receive."
"Most of the time, medicines are out of stock in the hospital and the town, which is a real recurring problem, especially because they are often essential for nephrology."
"Sometimes we run out of antibiotics and antihypertensives in the hospital for several days, not to mention the speciality medicines needed to manage dialysis patients."
"Medications are quite expensive in our region because they are imported from abroad, making them unaffordable for our patients. If any concrete action can be taken to mitigate the costs, it would be to produce them locally, here in our countries."

4. Health system-related factors

- **Limited resources,** limited national health budgets, high cost of care, and lack of universal health coverage.

   "You know, the issue at hand extends beyond the hospital. It is our healthcare system, operating within constrained budgets, which is making care provision difficult."
   "We can't even discuss the quality of care without universal health coverage."
   "Our country is committed to achieving universal health coverage, and we hope that this will improve the condition of our hospitals and the care provided to our patients."
   "The quality of healthcare is tied to the availability of resources; this is a fact. And regardless of our criticism of the hospital, the problem lies not only at its level."

- **Absence of a well-established patient referral system**, resulting in late referrals of patients in advanced stages of chronic kidney failure or to emergency for otherwise preventable complications.

   "Patients often seek medical consultation late, even when referred by the general practitioner for specialist advice, This is usually due to a lack of resources."
   "Currently, there is no clear channel or referral system in place, at least here. Most of the patients we receive are in advanced stages of the disease."

Thus, the interviewed doctors believe that various factors hinder social responsibility in their hospitals. They can be broadly summarised as follows:

- Understaffed healthcare system, as manifested in brain drain, and the lack of many medical and surgical specialities.
- The low number of hospitals and healthcare facilities.
- The cost of care and the absence of universal health coverage, as reflected in the shortage, high cost, and lack of local production of medicines.
- Issues with leadership and governance.
- Health financing challenges.

- Weak national information and research systems.
- Scarcity of information and communication technologies.

The shortage and high cost of medicines and the lack of universal health coverage were commonly reported by nephrologists from all regions. Nephrologists from sub-Saharan African countries reported these factors more frequently, along with the severe shortage of health professionals, particularly specialists. Likewise, the concept of "brain drain" and hospital overcrowding were also prevalent in most responses from sub-Saharan nephrologists.

African hospitals should cope with a large number of obstacles in order to provide quality care in the best possible conditions, in line with the dimensions of the social responsibility of hospitals.

- **The shortage of qualified and specialised healthcare professionals**, in this case nephrologists, vascular and urological surgeons, biologists, radiologists and resuscitators, whose collaboration is particularly useful in the management of kidney diseases.

On a global scale, there is a severe shortage of health professionals in 57 countries, 36 of them located in Africa. Developing countries are lacking 4 million health professionals. This crisis is worsened by the unequal distribution of health workers and the phenomenon of "brain drain". Nephrology experts around the world are increasingly concerned about the concept of "brain drain"[405,406,407,408,409].

For example, nephrology in the United States greatly benefits from foreign interns, many of whom do not return to their home countries. Consequently, these countries are losing valuable healthcare workforce. One reason for the reliance on foreign doctors is the diminishing appeal of nephrology as a specialty in the United States and other developed countries. At the same time, the demographics of kidney disease indicate a growing demand for nephrologists.

---

405 Parker MG, Pivert KA, Ibrahim T, Molitoris Recruiting the next generation of nephrologists. *Advances in Chronic Kidney Disease* 2013 July; 20(4): 326–335.
406 Squires D, Anderson C. US health care from a global perspective: spending, use of services, prices, and health in 13 countries. Commonwealth Fund 2015; 15: 1–16.
407 Poor health systems and lack of infrastructure paralyses health care in Africa. AFRIC Editorial; Dec. 2018. Available at: <https://afric.online/5626-poor-health-systems-and-lack-of-infrastructure-paralyses-health-care-in-africa/>.
408 Peters DH, Garg A, Bloom G et al. Poverty and access to health care in developing countries. *Annals of the New York Academy of Sciences* 2008; 1136(1): 161–171.
409 Kirigia JM, Barry SP. Health challenges in Africa and the way forward. *International Archives of Medicine* 2008; 1: 27.

In addition to the shortage of healthcare workers, there is a **lack of healthcare facilities, leading to overcrowding in the existing hospitals.**

- **The cost of healthcare and the lack of universal health coverage:** The cost, which includes medicines, surgeries, biological or radiological check-ups, consultations, and hospitalisations is generally considered unaffordable in resource-limited countries. This is because a large portion of healthcare expenses are is paid directly by individuals and families[410].
- **Leadership and governance:** The health sector in Africa is marked by weak leadership and ineffective organisation and management of health services, leading to an absence of vision and strategy. In addition, there is insufficient health legislation, limited community participation in planning and monitoring health services, weak inter-sectoral action, inequities in healthcare systems, and inefficiency in resource allocation and use, as reported by other authors[411,412].
- **Health financing in the African region** is characterized by low investment, lack of comprehensive health financing policies and strategic plans, weak financial management, inefficient resource use, and weak coordination of partner support[413].
- **Weak national health information and research systems**, along with the absence or inadequacy of kidney disease registry systems, hinders the understanding of dialysis outcomes. Furthermore, reliable estimates on kidney disease and treatment costs, including dialysis, in Africa are lacking[414].
- **The lack of information and communication technology** (e.g., low quality of broadband connection) limits the capacity of national health management information systems to generate, analyse, and disseminate information for decision making.

---

410   Ortiz-Prado E, Ponce J, Cornejo-Leon F et al. Analysis of health and drug access associated with the purchasing power of the Ecuadorian population. *Global Journal of Health Science* 2017; 9(1): 201–210.
411   *Strengthening health systems to improve health outcomes: WHO's framework for action.* Geneva: WHO; 2007.
412   Brinkerhoff DW, Bossert TJ. *Health governance: concepts, experience, and programming options.* Bethesda: Abt Associates Inc; 2008.
413   Kirigia JM, Barry SP. Health challenges in Africa and the way forward. *International Archives of Medicine* 2008; 1: 27.
414   Gething PW, Noor AM, Gikandi PW et al. Improving imperfect data from health management information systems in Africa using space-time geostatistics. *PLoS Med* 2006; 3: e271.

- **Reported abuses such as corruption** in the supply systems of medical technologies and products, unreliable supply chains, unaffordable prices, irrational use and a wide variation in quality and safety exist[415].

Regarding healthcare delivery, the lack of effective organisation and management of health services, alongside the aforementioned challenges, has resulted in a situation where 47 % of the population has no access to quality health services[416].

---

415 Carter M et al. Acute peritoneal dialysis treatment programs for countries of the East African community. *Blood Purification* 2012; 33: 149–152.
416 Kirigia JM, Barry SP. Health challenges in Africa and the way forward. *International Archives of Medicine* 2008; 1: 27.

Chapter 5: Ideas for enhancing hospital social responsibility in Africa

There are several models that can be used to address the various problems in the field of nephrology in Africa. These models mainly focus on screening, reducing risk factor, early diagnosis and treatment, and the importance of involving the government. They also include the dimensions of social responsibility in healthcare, such as adopting health policies, providing leadership and advocacy, securing financing, establishing public awareness programmes, and developing and allocating human resources. The World Kidney Day's awareness programmes provide an excellent platform for launching regional kidney screening programmes.

Nephrologists should collaborate with their local governments to establish sustainable programmes. In doing so, they should tailor experiences from other parts of the world to fit the cultural, environmental, and religious factors specific to their countries. Ultimately, it is believed that only Africans can solve the problems of Africa. Government funding, possibly in conjunction with public-private partnerships involving large local companies, could significantly contribute to the success of these programmes.

In our study, the nephrologists who responded to the questions about the factors hindering the social responsibility of their hospitals also proposed solutions for improving the situation. Their suggestions generally aligned with the factors influencing social responsibility they previously mentioned and discussed. However, their suggestions were mainly directed towards hospital managers and decision-makers of their healthcare systems. We categorised their suggestions into three parts as follows:

1. Recruiting and training the health workforce

- Establishing and improving local nephrologist training in order to increase their numbers and reduce the resulting brain drain. This is because, based on interviews with most doctors, a nephrologist trained in this specialty abroad might be more likely to settle and work in the host country. Moreover, local specialisation could better tailor the training to the local reality and epidemiology.

- Providing local training in various medical and surgical disciplines as well as in laboratory and imaging specialities. This also involves creating and strengthening a full technical platform at the hospital level.

  "To start, it's crucial for African countries be able to provide training for their own doctors and specialists. Many colleagues trained abroad end up staying there, and this is a reality that can't be ignored."
  "In order to expect an improvement in the current situation, we will need to train more doctors…"
  "There are countries with only one or two nephrologists. It is imperative that the training of nephrologists becomes a priority…"

- Giving special attention to continuing medical education. Universities and learned societies can play an important role in organising scientific nephrology events, facilitating group and institution subscriptions to the main specialty journals, creating local and/or regional journals, and encouraging the submission of high-quality, original work.

  "Continuing medical education is crucial. Universities, teaching hospitals, and scholarly societies have an important part to play in this."
  "Organising scientific events at least once or twice a year would be good for a start. We can't imagine quality care without continuing medical education."
  "Subscribing to one or two major Nephrology journals would also help us stay updated on the latest news in our specialty. This responsibility falls under the purview of the medical faculty and should be discussed with the specialised commissions within the institution."

- Training of doctors in effective communication: This aims to enhance patients' adherence to recommendations and foster their cooperation with the healthcare team throughout the care process.

  "Communication is essential for a strong doctor-patient relationship, especially when patients are dealing with complex, expensive, and chronic diseases. It should be incorporated into the medical programs or workshops."

- Recruiting and training the paramedical staff

  "It is essential to also recruit qualified nurses, especially in dialysis…"
  "The nephrologist also has a role to play in training their nursing staff…"

- Encouraging South-South cooperation for training and research purposes.

"We stand to gain significantly by collaborating and sharing experiences with neighbouring countries facing similar global challenges."
"It is time to consider collaboration between nephrologists, nephrology departments, and scholarly societies in various African countries."

2. Providing leadership and governance

The interviewed nephrologists stressed the importance of lobbying to make their voice heard by decision-makers, with the aim to:

- Prioritise kidney disease and increase the budget allocated to it.
- Improve the availability of medicines needed for treating kidney patients at affordable prices.
- Promote local production of medicines and dialysis products through investment and favourable fiscal measures.
- Authorise, when marketing generic medicines, only molecules with controlled bio-equivalence studies.

"Nephrologists need to engage in lobbying in order to be heard by decision-makers…"
"Kidney disease should be seen as a public health priority, and it is up to us, nephrologists, to advocate for this cause with the policy makers…"
"When kidney diseases are given priority, we can then hopefully secure an increase in the budget for managing these diseases and improve the availability of medicines. We should also focus on local production. We should stop depending on the rest of the world and develop our local pharmaceutical industry."
"The local production of medicines and equipment should be more seriously considered if we want to get out of this situation…"
"Generic medicines are also a solution for reducing costs and widening access to care… It is, however, necessary to ensure that these molecules have bio-equivalence studies."
"Generic medicines can be a solution, for sure, but we still need to have confidence in the molecules being commercialised."

In addition, the interviewed nephrologists emphasised the importance of advocating for kidney disease by suggesting that nephrology practitioners should:

- Take on roles of responsibility within their healthcare facilities. This would help bring attention to the challenges of managing kidney disease, which are often overlooked by the managers of these institutions.
- Establish local professional associations to create a solid foundation with scientific and moral credibility.

- Promote research efforts and establish national registers for kidney disease in order to develop a reliable information system and gain a better understanding of local epidemiology and, consequently. This will help identify actual human and logistical requirements.

    "It is also important to promote research in our African context. This will help us gain a better understanding of our local and regional epidemiology and establish registries, as is done in developed countries. When discussing with decision-makers and trying to convince them, it's crucial to present accurate information supported with figures ."
    "We also need learned societies to advocate for the specialty before decision-makers."

- Implementing and generalising universal health coverage, which is a key part of equitable access to quality care.

    "There is no possibility for providing quality care or fulfilling hospital social responsibility without implementing and generalising universal health coverage. This is the first step to take in order to improve the current situation."
    "Universal health coverage could be a solution…"

3. Strengthening infrastructure and logistics

- Increasing the number of pertinent quality care facilities

    "In addition to nephrologists, we need to increase the number and quality of hospital structures in order to improve access to care."
    "It is crucial to improve the infrastructure and equipment of the hospitals where we work, and to consider expanding the number of healthcare facilities."

The suggestions provided by the participating doctors focussed on several key areas: The need for broader health coverage, local production of affordable medicines, for an increase in the number of healthcare facilities and professionals, especially specialists, and to address the issue of brain drain. They also emphasised the importance of good governance and the value of lobbying to persuade decision-makers to support their proposals.

In North Africa, for example, the participating nephrologists mainly recommended reasonably priced medicine (76.6 %), an increase in the number of healthcare facilities to accommodate the large number of patients (46.6 %), and the establishment of universal health coverage (39.9 %).

Doctors in sub-Saharan Africa proposed an increase in the number of medical and paramedical teams, especially specialists (80 %–100 %), local production of affordable and accessible medicines, introduction of universal health coverage (66.6 %–100 %), and action against brain drain (33.3 %–80 %).

It is important to note that all these suggestions can be further discussed and developed within the framework of the WHO's healthcare systems[417,418,419] which includes:

1. Service delivery: Management, infrastructure, quality and safety, and provision of care.
2. Health workforce: Human resources.
3. Information systems: Population-based information and surveillance systems and facilities, global tools and standards.
4. Medical products, vaccines and technologies: Norms, standards, policies, reliable supply, equitable access, and quality.
5. Financing: National health financing policies, health expenditure tools and data, and costing.
6. Leadership and governance: Health sector policies, harmonisation and alignment, monitoring and regulation.

1. Service delivery:

– Management at the hospital level

Managing commitment is one of the most important components of hospital social responsibility, as demonstrated by Kakabadse and Rozuel[420] in a French hospital. While studying the social responsibility of five private hospitals in Bangalore, India, Rohini also underscored the contribution of hospital managers to making their hospitals socially responsible. It is, therefore, crucial to improve the organisation, fund management, and quality of services of hospitals to enhance their social responsibility. However, this places a heavy burden on managers, as indicated in African reports. These reports also pointed out that highly trained managers in Africa are rare in Africa, while funding is often insufficient and existing managers are overwhelmed by multiple tasks. For

---

417 *Strengthening health systems to improve health outcomes: WHO's framework for action.* Geneva: WHO; 2007.
418 Brinkerhoff DW, Bossert TJ. *Health governance: Concepts, experience, and programming options.* Bethesda: Abt Associates Inc; 2008.
419 Monitoring the building blocks of health systems: a handbook of indicators and their measurement strategies. Available at: <http://www.who.int/healthinfo/systems/monitoring/en/>.
420 Kakabadse N, Rozuel C. Meaning of corporate social responsibility in a local French hospital: a case study. *Society and Business Review* 2006; 1: 77–96.

example, they need to ensure access to services, engage a wide range of healthcare providers, ensure quality, and ensure that health priorities are met. Therefore, it is essential to provide manager training and support through trained and motivated administrative staff.

– Strategies for improving healthcare services: Improving the care process

Quality control, and therefore the proper allocation of resources, has become a central issue in the management of healthcare systems. Multiple tools are used to monitor the levels of care and enhance its quality. Clinical audit is one of the most popular and widely used among these tools. In the field of clinical nephrology, this method has proven its effectiveness in addressing various health issues such as hypertension and mineral metabolism control. However, it is still necessary to increase awareness about clinical audit and encourage its consistent application at both national and local levels. This will allow it to become an integral part of the expertise of each healthcare provider, alongside other quality improvement techniques[421].

– Infrastructure

Nephrology and dialysis departments/units need to be established and equipped according to the strategies adopted in recent years by several African countries to address health infrastructure challenges. Decentralisation initiatives are examples of these strategies, which contributed to a more equitable distribution of health centres to meet local needs. Also, many countries experienced improvements in healthcare delivery and through the increased involvement of non-state healthcare providers such as non-profit and faith-based organisations[422]. Investing in improved nephrology infrastructure planning in the following areas could yield significant benefits: decentralising kidney healthcare with realistic and tailored services and equipment, especially in remote areas; providing appropriate levels of training for healthcare professionals in these centres; implementing innovative, cost-effective health services through e-health technology; and deploying low-cost, mobile medical equipment that can be used across different decentralised centres.

---

421 Esposito P, Dal Canton A. Clinical audit, a valuable tool to improve quality of care: general methodology and applications in nephrology. *World Journal of Nephrology* 2014; 3(4): 249–255.

422 Investir dans la santé en Afrique. Harmonisation pour la santé en Afrique. OMS; 2011. Available at: <https://www.who.int/pmnch/media/membernews/2011/investir_sante_afrique.pdf?ua=1>.

Other infrastructure improvements including better communication networks and access to water and sanitation would also public health. Collaborative efforts between health ministries and other ministries through multi-sectoral approaches are also expected to have direct beneficial effects on community health, such as improvements in water, sanitation, and transportation.

– Patient data protection

As mentioned earlier, protecting patient data relies on a robust archiving system. Moreover, the WHO recommends that healthcare records personnel must uphold confidentiality and take responsibility for preventing unauthorised access to those records[423].

2. The health workforce (caregivers)

– Nephrologists
– More nephrologists should be trained to comply with the standards set by learned societies and to address the kidney healthcare needs of African populations.
– Emphasis should be placed on practical clinical training, preferably within the physician's own region. This approach will increase the relevance and effectiveness of the training while reducing costs and the risk of "brain drain".
– It is important to assess the value of e-learning needs in improving the knowledge and skills of health professionals in managing kidney diseases, including their impact on healthcare inequities.
– In the short term, training programmes should focus on raising awareness and supporting prevention. In the medium term, they should aim to enhance the quality of therapeutic interventions. In the long term, they should facilitate participation in advocacy and governance to achieve comprehensive management of kidney patients through collaboration between industry, research groups, clinical experts, and patient groups[424,425].

---

423 Mathebeni-Bokwe P. Management of medical records for healthcare service delivery at the Victoria Public Hospital in the Eastern Cape Province: South Africa (thesis). Alice (South Africa): Fort Hare univ.; 2015. Available at: <https://pdfs.semanticscholar.org/e888/2023a43f5266449c6eed35f092f02e47163f.pdf>.
424 Mullan F, Frehywot S, Omaswa F et al. Medical schools in sub-Saharan Africa. *Lancet* 2011; 377: 1113–1121.
425 Feehally J, Brusselmans A, Finkelstein FO et al. Improving global health: measuring the success of capacity building outreach programs: a view from the International Society of Nephrology. *Kidney International* 2016; 6: 42–51.

– Paramedical staff (nurses and technicians)

Training programmes for paramedical staff should emphasise practical and relevant lessons on dealing with common pathologies[426,427,428].

- Encouraging paramedical staff to stay in their local areas and utilise their new skills instead of migrating to larger cities or abroad.
- Training programmes, like those provided by the International Society of Nephrology, should promote the use of locally available equipment and expertise instead of introducing complex technical procedures that require external expertise. The latter can lead to a drain of funds to foreign providers instead of supporting the local economy.
- Health auxiliaries and the nursing aids

Investing in the education of the local population to recruit and train motivated health workers, such as health auxiliaries and the nursing aids, will benefit the entire community and improve healthcare equity.

It is essential, in the context of the Strategy on Human Resources for Universal Access to Health and Universal Health Coverage approved by the 29th Pan American Health Conference in 2017, to consider the interests, motivations, and working conditions required for health workforce in underserved areas with the aim of attracting and retaining human resources in those areas. For example, financial incentives for health workforce might be worth considering for assignments in remote areas.

3. Information

Sound decision making, which helps in allocating resources appropriately and in eliminating inequalities in care delivery, requires continued access to data and research. Registers provide this important service. It is imperative that all countries allocate resources to data collection and quality monitoring. In addition to standard treatment-related parameters, registers must compile data

---

426 Okel J, Okpechi IG, Qarni B, et al. Nephrology training curriculum and implications for optimal kidney care in the developing world. *Clinical Nephrology* 2016; 86: 110–113.

427 Anderson JE, Torres JR, Bitter DC et al. Role of physician assistants in dialysis units and nephrology. *American Journal of Kidney Diseases* 1999; 33: 647–651.

428 Steinman TI. Nephrology workforce shortfall: solutions are needed. *American Journal of Kidney Diseases* 1999; 33: 798–800.

on parameters of discrimination (e.g., background, education, gender, ethnicity, migrant status, place of residence) as well as comorbidities to ensure that the system does not exacerbate inequities.

4. Providing medical products: The availability of medicines, cost control, equity of treatment

Generic medicines offer a promising solution in the African context. According to the Food and Drug Administration (FDA), they are medications that have the same effectiveness and safety properties as their branded counterparts but at more affordable prices. Several European studies have proven these claims, allowing health authorities to adopt generic medicines as a cost-saving measure without compromising care. Prescribing high-quality generics conserves significant resources for patients and healthcare systems, which is particularly important in sub-Saharan Africa, where the healthcare sector is underfunded, and out-of-pocket payments are widespread.

The role played by the WHO and other international agencies in ensuring the supply of quality generic medicines for diseases such as malaria, Tuberculosis, and HIV has made a positive impact on patient outcomes. Extending this process to other essential medicines, particularly for non-communicable diseases such as hypertension and diabetes, would likely have similar outcome. Additionally, strict regulation, including proven medicine bio-equivalence, would increase doctors' confidence in prescribing generic medicines.

This can be achieved through quality assurance programmes, which are mandatory for local generic manufacturers, and through the legal provision of bio-equivalence data and standards[429,430].

Furthermore, it is important to establish a pan-African database for organ transplantation. This would be valuable if Africa decides to negotiate for more affordable immunosuppressive medicines collectively.

Creating centres of excellence across the continent to enhance local training and attract international support is also crucial. The first step would involve

---

429   Fadare JO, Adeoti AO, Desalu OO et al. The prescribing of generic medicines in Nigeria: knowledge, perceptions and attitudes of physicians. *Expert Review of Pharmacoeconomics & Outcomes Research* 2016; 16(5): 639–650.
430   t Hoen EF, Hogerzeil HV, Quick JD. A quiet revolution in global public health: the World Health Organization's prequalification of medicines programme. *Journal of Public Health Policy* 2014; 35(2): 137–161.

consolidating all ongoing efforts, documenting and monitoring them, and using the information to develop comprehensive programmes for these centres.

- Local production of medicines

There is an urgent need to increase doctors' confidence in generic medicines produced by local manufacturers and to improve the prescribing of international non-proprietary names (INNs) in general. This will benefit local manufacturers as well as patients and healthcare systems.

- Controlling healthcare costs

The control or reduction of the healthcare costs can be achieved through the following measures:

- Definition of clear indications for treatments use.
- Implementation of preventive measures such as controlling infections, high blood pressure, and type 2 diabetes to reduce the incidence of end-stage kidney disease. This may also include early detection interventions to prevent the progression of advanced kidney disease requiring dialysis, which could alleviate excessive use of healthcare resources.
- Efforts to reduce the costs of consumables, for example, by combining purchase agreements between suppliers to aggregate demand or addressing supply monopolies.
- At the level of health authorities and health policymakers, it is important to establish clear strategies based on a thorough assessment of the needs and opportunities for kidney disease care, including replacement therapy. In some countries, such as Thailand, where not all patients can afford dialysis, recommendations based on transparent decision making are being adopted to optimise the use of this limited resource. For example, peritoneal dialysis is freely offered to patients, but those who refuse this treatment option do not receive financial support. In South African public hospitals, dialysis is only offered to eligible patients willing to be transplanted when a kidney transplant is available[431].

---

431 Van Biesen W, Jha V, Abu-Alfa AK. Considerations on equity in management of end-stage kidney disease in low- and middle-income countries. *Kidney International Supplements*. 2020; 10: e63–e71.

- Local manufacturing of dialysis products and consumables can reduce the overall cost of dialysis, prevent economic resources from going to other countries, and create local job opportunities.
- **Equity of healthcare delivery:** Developing locally appropriate financing models is essential to ensure that there are no out-of-pocket expenses for patients receiving replacement therapy. Successful models implemented in middle- and low-income countries like Colombia and Thailand[432,433] have shown that allocating sufficient funds to healthcare services is more of a "political" decision than a financial one, with a higher proportion of GDP being allocated to public health. For instance, Colombia has achieved universal access to dialysis despite having a low GDP. Consequently, out-of-pocket spending on replacement therapy is currently low.
- **Accessibility of health care:** Improving this accessibility can be facilitated through the following measures:
- Implementing a decentralised approach to kidney failure treatment, especially in rural areas, by establishing health facilities that offer nephrology care in these areas.
- Subsidising the cost of health services in rural areas, although it may be unachievable in the African region, as charges in rural areas are already twice as low as in urban areas[434].
- Embracing new technologies like telemedicine to ensure equitable dissemination of knowledge among health professionals and to provide quality care and prevention activities.

When developing e-health care schemes, it is important to ensure that the tools meet the real needs of the different stakeholders instead of creating new needs. These tools should reach those with limited access to health services to prevent further disadvantages.

---

432 Lopera-Medina MM. *Utilización de servicios de salud por enfermedades catastró cas o de alto costo en Antioquia. La Revista Gerencia y Políticas de Salud* 2017; 16 (32): 120–137.
433 Chuengsaman P, Kasemsup V. PD first policy: Thailand's response to the challenge of meeting the needs of patients with end-stage renal disease. *Seminars in Nephrology* 2017; 37: 287–295.
434 Osborn R, Squires D, Doty MM et al. In New survey of eleven countries, US adults still struggle with access to and affordability of health care. *Health Affairs* 2016; 35(12): 2327–2336.

Finally, it is worth noting that existing evidence on e-health applications for kidney patients is inconclusive[435,436,437,438,439].

5. Securing financing: Funds and investments

– Government investment in the healthcare sector

The promotion of kidney disease management requires a strong healthcare system with adequate funding. Indeed, African health authorities should lobby the international community and the WHO for funding to support health promotion. Investments in the healthcare sector should focus on strengthening programmes related to social welfare, nutrition? and catastrophic diseases, managed by the Ministries of Health and other relevant bodies. These investments aim to ensure the implementation of public health policies that guarantee access to quality healthcare services and medicines.

Additionally, studies have shown that public policies focussing on education and health services can lead to long-term improvements in the overall health of the population[440,441].

---

435 Calvillo-Arbizu J, Roa-Romero LM, Estudillo-Valderrama MA et al. User- centred design for developing e-Health system for renal patients at home (AppNephro). *International Journal of Medical Informatics* 2019;125:47–54.

436 Singh K, Diamantidis CJ, Ramani S et al. Patients' and nephrologists' evaluation of patient-facing smartphone apps for CKD. *Clinical Journal of the American Society of Nephrology* 2019; 14: 523–529.

437 Bonner A, Gillespie K, Campbell KL et al. Evaluating the prevalence and opportunity for technology use in chronic kidney disease patients: a cross-sectional study. *BMC Nephrology* 2018; 19: 28.

438 Topf JM, Hiremath S. Got CKD? There's an app for that! *Clinical Journal of the American Society of Nephrology* 2019; 14: 491–492.

439 Stenberg K, Hanssen O, Edejer TT et al. Financing transformative health systems towards achievement of the health Sustainable Development Goals: a model for projected resource needs in 67 low-income and middle-income countries. *Lancet Global Health* 2017;5:e875–e877.

440 Ortiz-Prado E, Ponce J, Cornejo-Leon F et al. Analysis of health and drug access associated with the purchasing power of the Ecuadorian population. *Global Journal of Health Science* 2017; 9(1): 201–210.

441 Revicki DA. *Gut* 2004; 53(Suppl IV): iv40–iv44.

6. Providing leadership and governance (at the level of health authorities in African regions and countries)

Socially responsible health structures require strong leadership to define the strategic vision and mobilise efforts towards its realisation. It also requires adequate governance to ensure the effective use of resources and tangible outcomes that achieve the defined objectives. This involves directing and engaging partners and staff, facilitating change, and improving the quality of health services through effective, innovative, and accountable allocation of staff and other resources[442].

In low-income countries, particularly in Africa, there is currently a lack of leadership and governance capacity in both the private and public sectors. Therefore, there is a need to better define competencies, roles, and responsibilities with a systematic focus on determining the most effective interventions. These countries should then proceed with the implementation of an action plan to develop leadership and governance capacity, including the possibility of international assistance in this field.

In addition to the proposed elements of the healthcare system, breaking down the barriers between different health sectors and establishing public-private partnerships are becoming increasingly necessary. Moreover, improving people's living standards remains crucial. Therefore, government health policies should be developed in conjunction with economic strategies to improve the quality of life of African populations.

It is widely recognised that improvements in water and sanitation infrastructure highly contribute to population health. Safe water and sanitation play a significant role in creating a healthier environment, as discussed in medical literature. Better water and sanitation are linked to reduced exposure to pathogens[443].

Furthermore, it is important to encourage investment in both the healthcare sector and human capital through education and training. In addition, access to healthcare should be complemented by access to adequate food, water, sanitation, and education[444]. Besides, health policies play a key role in reducing health disparities

---

442 Améliorer le leadership et la gestion sanitaire: Rapport d'une consultation internationale sur le renforcement du leadership et de la gestion dans les pays à faible revenu. OMS; 2007. Available at: <https://www.who.int/management/working_paper_10_fr_opt.pdf>.
443 Briscoe J, Feachem R, Rahaman M. *Evaluating health impact: water supply, sanitation and hygiene education*. Ottawa: International Development Research Centre; 1986.
444 Barrera A. The role of maternal schooling and its interaction with public health programs in child health production. *Journal of Development Economics* 1990; 32: 69–92.

between rural and urban areas, particularly in improving the health status of rural populations.

At another level, addressing gender disparities is also crucial. Women's education and socio-economic empowerment are essential for better health outcomes. A key action for positive change is improving women's access to education, especially in the African region. Therefore, policymakers should allocate more resources to enhance girls' access to schools. Yet, this empowerment will be incomplete unless women are also allowed to fully participate in the labour market and benefit from their own work[445].

In summary, social responsibility in healthcare necessitates the implementation of measures that will directly impact the quality and equity of healthcare delivery. This cannot be achieved without strengthening the various components of healthcare systems (service delivery, information systems, human resources, medical products and technologies, financing, leadership, and governance), along with improvements in people's standard of living, while considering the social determinants of health. These actions require a structured partnership between different stakeholders, including political actors, at the local level of a region or country. This partnership should be guided by identified needs to enhance accessibility and equity in quality care. Only then can our hospitals be considered socially responsible (Figure 15).

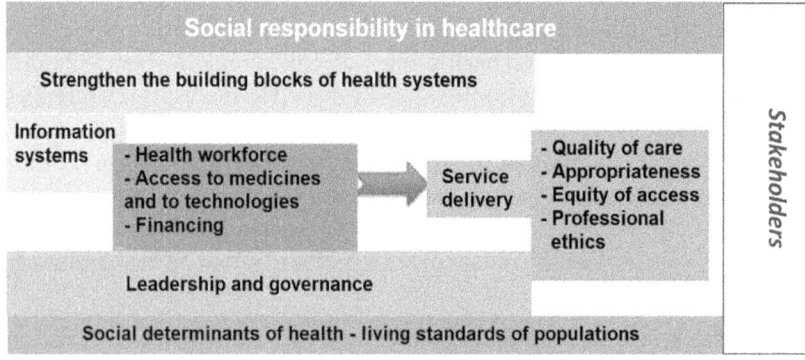

Figure 15: Social responsibility in healthcare: A global concept

---

445 A Summary of the Report of the Commission on Women's Health in the African Region. World Health Organization, Regional office for Africa; 2012.

Conclusion

Based on principles of quality, efficiency, pertinence, and equity, hospital social responsibility is widely seen as a necessary action for improving patient care in most developed countries. Our study showed that only a small proportion of patients had a positive perception of hospital social responsibility. While patients were generally satisfied with the therapeutic management and involvement of caregivers, they expressed dissatisfaction with the hospital environment, general conditions, accessibility, and equity of care. The study also found a significant positive correlation between health coverage, a country's income level, public spending on health and education, and patients' perceptions of hospital social responsibility.

Regarding doctors, most of them felt that their hospitals were not socially responsible. They identified various factors hindering the social responsibility of African hospitals, such as a shortage of healthcare professionals, poor governance, inadequate infrastructure, as well as issues related to the healthcare system itself, including small national budgets, high cost of care, and lack of health coverage.

Our study emphasised the importance of hospital governance and management by involving different stakeholders to enhance the social responsibility of hospitals and overall care delivery. This is a new governance approach to create organisational value through performance, compliance, and accountability.

Although not fully representative of all kidney patients and nephrologists, the perceptions and concerns of our participants offer valuable insights for health authorities into how hospitals and kidney disease management in Africa are perceived. This information can be instrumental for decision-makers, influencing healthcare policies, improving the performance of our healthcare systems, and fostering socially responsible actions.

However, there are several limitations to our study. The results obtained should be interpreted with caution because the participants (patients and nephrologists) do not represent all stakeholders of the healthcare system or all African countries. Additionally, local teams performed translations of questionnaires into indigenous dialects, and we were unable to verify the accuracy of these translations. Also, the questionnaires were only sent to motivated doctors who had agreed to participate in the study, which may have introduced a selection bias in our recruitment method. Moreover, our survey did not investigate the impact of patients' clinical and para-clinical data, nor did it assess possible links between this data and perceptions of hospital social responsibility. More research in this field is needed before the study's results can be generalised. It would be valuable to conduct surveys with adequate representation of patients, nephrologists, and healthcare system decision-makers across the continent.

References

A Review of Corporate Social Responsibility for Health in Africa. United States Agency for International Development; Dec. 2014. Disponible: <http://www.africanstrategies4health.com/resources.aspx>.

A Summary of the Report of the Commission on Women's Health in the African Region. World Health Organization, Regional office for Africa; 2012.

Abd ElHafeez S, Bolignano D, D'Arrigo G et al. Prevalence and burden of chronic kidney disease among the general population and high-risk groups in Africa: a systematic review. *BMJ Open* 2018; 8: e015069.

Abraham KA, Thompson EB, Bodger K et al. Inequalities in outcomes of acute kidney injury in England. *QJM* 2012; 105: 729–740.

Abreu R, David F, Crowther D. Corporate social responsibility is urgently needed in health care. *Social Responsibility Journal* 2005; 1(3/4): 225–240.

Abu-aisha H, Elamin S. Peritoneal dialysis in Africa. *Peritoneal Dialysis International: Journal of the International Society for Peritoneal Dialysis* 2010; 30: 23–28.

Ackoundou-Nguessan C, Gnionsahe A, Guie M et al. High failure rate for first arterio-venous fistula for patients starting hemodialysis treatment: a report from Ivory Coast. *Saudi Journal of Kidney Diseases and Transplantation* 2008; 19: 384e8.

Acquier A, Gond JP. Aux sources de la responsabilité sociale de l'entreprise: relecture et analyse d'un ouvrage fondateur: Social responsabilities of the businnessman d'Howard Bowen, 1953, Finance-Contrôle- Stratégie 2007; 10(2): 5–35.

Addendum for the plan of action and budget 2008–2012. World Health Organization and African Programme for Onchocerciasis Control (APOC). WHO; 2008. Disponible: <https://apps.who.int/iris/handle/10665/274421/browse?authority=Strategic+Planning&type=mesh>.

Adejumo OA, Akinbodewa AA, Ogunleye A et al. Cost implication of inpatient care of chronic kidney disease patients in a tertiary hospital in Southwest Nigeria. *Saudi Journal of Kidney Diseases and Transplantation* 2020; 31: 209–214.

AFDB. "The Middle of the Pyramid, Dynamics of the Middle class in Africa", Mar. 2011.

Afrique subsaharienne. Un changement de cap s'impose. coll. « Perspectives économiques régionales », Fond monétaire international; avr. 2016.

Alderson K, Meale E. Industries extractives – Vue d'ensemble [archive]. Banque mondiale; 15 Sept. 2015.

Alkhodair AA, Aleisa SN, Alghamdi MA. Satisfaction level among nephrologists towards chronic kidney disease patients referred from Primary Health Care System. *The Egyptian Journal of Hospital Medicine* 2018; 70(10): 1801–1807.

Almutairi OO, Alqarni AA, Alzahrani SA et al. Patients' satisfaction with Health Care Services in Southern Saudi Arabia. *The Egyptian Journal of Hospital Medicine* 2018; 72(1): 3857–3860.

Améliorer le leadership et la gestion sanitaire. Rapport d'une consultation internationale sur le renforcement du leadership et de la gestion dans les pays à faible revenu. OMS; 2007. Disponible: <https://www.who.int/management/working_paper_10_fr_opt.pdf>.

Amoran OE, Omokhodion FO, Dairo MD et al. Job satisfaction among primary health care workers in three selected local government areas in southwest Nigeria. *Nigerian Journal of Medicine* 2005; 14: 195–199.

Anderson JE, Torres JR, Bitter DC et al. Role of physician assistants in dialysis units and nephrology. *American Journal of Kidney Diseases* 1999; 33: 647–651.

Appauvrissement et dégradation des terres et des eaux: menace grandissante pour la sécurité alimentaire. FAO; 28 Nov. 2011.

Arendse C, Okpechi I, Swanepoel C. Acute dialysis in HIV-positive patients in Cape Town, South Africa. *Nephrology* 2011; 16: 39–44.

Arije A, Kadiri S, Akinkugbe O. The viability of hemodialysis as a treatment option for renal failure in a developing economy. *African Journal of Medicine and Medical Sciences* 2000; 29: 311–314.

Ashish K, Jha E, Orav J et al. Patients' perception of hospital care in the United States. *New England Journal of Medicine* 2008; 359: 1921–1931.

Assounga AG, Assambo-Kielim C, Mafoua A, Moyenm G, Nzingoula S. Etiology and outcome of acute renal failure in children in Congo-Brazzaville. *Saudi Journal of Kidney Diseases and Transplantation* 2000; 11: 40–43.

Atlas des statistiques sanitaires africaines 2016. Analyse de la situation sanitaire de la Région africaine. Observatoire africain de la santé, Organisation mondiale de la Santé, Bureau régional de l'Afrique OMS (2017), Financement de l'accès universel à l'eau, l'assainissement et l'hygiène dans le cadre des objectifs de développement durable. Rapport d'analyse et d'évaluations globales de l'assainissement et de l'eau potable (GLAAS) 2017 de l'ONU-Eau. Genève: Organisation mondiale de la Santé; 2017.

Background, principles and application. Paris: UNESCO Publishing; 2009.

Bamgboye EL, Mabayoje MO, Odutola TA, Mabadeje AF. Acute renal failure at the Lagos University Teaching Hospital: a 10-year review. *Renal Failure* 1993; 15: 77–80.

Barrera A. The role of maternal schooling and its interaction with public health programs in child health production. *Journal of Development Economics* 1990; 32: 69–92.

Barsoum RS, Khalil SS, Arogundade FA. Fifty years of dialysis in Africa: challenges and progress. *American Journal of Kidney Diseases* 2015; 65(3): 502–512.

Barsoum RS. History of dialysis in Africa. In Ing TS, Rahman MA, Kjellstrand CM, ed., *Dialysis: history, development and promise*. Singapore: World Scientific Publishing Co.; 2012. pp. 599–610.

Beauchamp TL, Childress JF. *Principles of biomedical ethics*. 7th ed. Oxford: Oxford University Press; 2013.

Benghanem Gharbi M. et al. Prevalence of chronic kidney disease and associated risk factors: first results from a population based screening program in Morocco (MAREMAR). *Journal of the American Society of Nephrology* 2012; 23: 178A.

Berrou JP, Gondard-Delcroix C. Dynamique des réseaux sociaux et résilience socio-économique des micro-entrepreneurs informels en milieu urbain africain. *Mondes en développement*. 2011; 4(156): 73–88.

Bhuiyan A. Community health providers and their social responsibility. *International Journal of Gynecology & Obstetrics* 2009; 107: S. 128.

Bieber B et al. Two-times weekly hemodialysis in China: frequency, associated patient and treatment characteristics and Quality of Life in the China Dialysis Outcomes and Practice Patterns study. *Nephrology Dialysis Transplantation* 2014; 29:1770–7.

Blake PG. PD growth in the developing world. *Peritoneal Dialysis International* 2010; 30: 5–6.

Blane D et al. Disease etiology and materialist explanations of socioeconomic mortality differentials. *European Journal of Public Health* 1997; 7: 385–391.

Boelen C, Défis et opportunités des partenariats pour le développement de la santé. Bases factuelles et information à l'appui des politiques Département de Prestation des services de santé. WHO; 2001.

Boelen C, Heck JE & World Health Organization. Division of Development of Human Resources for Health. In: Charles Boelen et Jeffery E. Heck, ed., *Définir et mesurer la responsabilité sociale des facultés de médecine*. Genève: Organisation mondiale de la Santé; 2000. Disponible: <https://apps.who.int/iris/handle/10665/66532>.

Boelen C, Heck JE & World Health Organization. Division of Development of Human Resources for Health. Définir et mesurer la responsabilité sociale des facultés de médecine / Charles Boelen et Jeffery E. Heck. Genève: Organisation mondiale de la Santé; 2000. Disponible: <https://apps.who.int/iris/handle/10665/66532>

Boelen C. Interlinking medical practice and medical education. Prospects for international action. In: Walton H, ed., *Proceedings of the world summit on medical education*. Medical Education, 1994, suppl. 1, 28: 82–85.

Boelen C. Consensus Mondial sur la Responsabilité Sociale des Facultés de Médecine. *Santé publique* 2011; 23(3): 247–250.

Bonner A, Gillespie K, Campbell KL et al. Evaluating the prevalence and opportunity for technology use in chronic kidney disease patients: a cross-sectional study. *BMC Nephrology* 2018; 19: 28.

Bosho C, Gray B. The relationships between service quality, customer satisfaction and buying intentions in the private hospital industry. *South African Journal of Business Management* 2004; 35(4): 27–37.

Bowen HR. *Social responsibilities of the businessman*. New York: Harper; 1953.

Brandão C et al. Social responsibility: a new paradigm of hospital governance?. *Health Care Analysis* 2013; 21(4): 390–402.

Brewer KM. Corporate social responsibility in the pharmaceutical industry – why it matters from business, bioethical and social perspectives (Thesis). Winston-Salem (NC): WAKE FOREST Univ., 2014.

Briesacher BA, Andrade SE, Fouayzi H et al. Medication adherence and use of generic drug therapies. *The American Journal of Managed Care* 2009; 15(7): 450–456.

Brinkerhoff DW, Bossert TJ. *Health governance: concepts, experience, and programming options*. Bethesda: Abt Associates Inc; 2008.

Briscoe J, Feachem R, Rahaman M. *Evaluating health impact: water supply, sanitation and hygiene education*. Ottawa: International Development Research Centre; 1986.

Brunel S, L'Afrique est-elle si bien partie? éd. *sciences humaines*; Oct. 2014.

Brunet-Jailly. *Innover dans les systèmes de santé; expériences d' Afrique de l'Ouest*. Paris: Karthala, 1997: 257–270.

Business in development: AngloGold Ashanti and The Global Fund in Ghana. The United Kingdom Department for International Development (DFID) – Johns Hopkins Center for Communication Programs (CCP); 2017. Disponible: <https://www.icmm.com/document/4673>.

Callegari J,·Antwi SB. Peritoneal dialysis as a mode of treatment for acute kidney injury in sub-Saharan Africa. *Blood Purification* 2013; 36: 226–230.

Calvillo-Arbizu J, Roa-Romero LM, Estudillo-Valderrama MA et al. User-centred design for developing e-Health system for renal patients at home (AppNephro). *International Journal of Medical Informatics* 2019; 125: 47–54.

Cameron A, Mantel-Teeuwisse AK, Leufkens HG. Switching from originator brand medicines to generic equivalents in selected developing countries: how much could be saved? *Value in Health. The Journal of the International Society for Pharmacoeconomics and Outcomes Research* 2012; 15(5): 664–73.

Caramel L. Éducation: l'Afrique toujours dans le peloton de queue. *Le Monde* 9 avr. 2015.

Carter M et al. Acute peritoneal dialysis treatment programs for countries of the East African community. *Blood Purification* 2012; 33: 149–152.

Cauli M, Boelen C, Ladner J. et al. Dictionnaire francophone de la responsabilité sociale en santé. Presses universitaires de Rouen et du Havre; 2019.

CEA, Commission de l'Union africaine et FNUAP: « Déclaration d'Addis-Abeba sur la population et le développement après 2014 ». Addis-Abeba (Éthiopie); 2013. Disponible: <www.unfpa.org/sites/de- fault/ les/event-pdf/declaration-nal-e1351225.pdf>.

CEA, Union africaine, Groupe de la Banque africaine de développement et Programme des Nations Unies pour le développement: Rapport sur les OMD 2014: Évaluation des progrès accomplis en Afrique dans la réalisation des objectifs du Millénaire pour le développement. Addis–Abeba; 2014. Disponible: <www.uneca.org/sites/default/les/PublicationFiles/2014_mdg_report. pdf>.

Chodzaza E, Bultemeier K. Service providers' perception of the quality of emergency obsteric care provided and factors identified which affect the provision of quality care. *Malawi Medical Journal* 2010; 22(4): 104–11.

Chrétien JP. *Le défi de l'ethnisme. Rwanda et Burundi: 1990 – 1996 (fiche bibliographique du centre de documentation du CNRS)*. Paris: éd. Karthala; 1997.

Chrétien JP, Mukuri M. *Burundi, la fracture identitaire: logiques de violence et certitudes ethniques, 1993–1996*. Paris: éd. Karthala; 2002.

Chuengsaman P, Kasemsup V. PD first policy: Thailand's response to the challenge of meeting the needs of patients with end-stage renal disease. *Seminars in Nephrology* 2017; 37: 287–295.

Closing the gap in health equity through action on the social determinants of health. Geneva: World Health Organization Commission on Social Determinants on Health. WHO; 2008. Disponible: <http://www.who.int/social_determinants/thecommission/finalre-port/en/index.html>.

Codreanu I, Perico N, Sharma SK et al. Prevention programmes of progressive renal disease in developing nations. *Nephrology* 2006; 11: 321–328.

Collins SK. Corporate social responsibility and the future health care manager. *The Health Care Manager* 2010; 29(4): 339–345.

Composition des régions macrogéographiques (continentales), composantes géographiques des régions et composition de groupements sélectionnés économiques et d'autres groupements. [archive]. Organisation des Nations unies; 2015.

Conradie A, Duys R, Forget P et al. Barriers to clinical research in Africa: a quantitative and qualitative survey of clinical researchers in 27 African countries. *British Journal of Anaesthesia* 2018; 121(4): 813e821.

Coresh J et al. Prevalence of chronic kidney disease in the United States. *JAMA* 2007; 298(17): 2038–2047.

Cunningham CT, Quan H, Hemmelgarn B et al. Exploring physician specialist response rates to web-based surveys. *BMC Medical Research Methodology* 2015; 15: 32.

D'Almeida-Topor H. L'Afrique du xxe siècle à nos jours. éd. Armand Colin. coll. « U »; 2013.

De la Moussaye E, Jacquemot P. Politique de santé, les trois options stratégiques. *Afrique contemporaine* 1993: 166: 15–26.

Dechambenoit G. Access to health care in sub-Saharan Africa. *Surgical Neurology International* 2016; 7: 108.

Définition de « responsabilité ». Disponible: <https://www.lalanguefrancaise.com/dictionnaire/definition-responsabilite/>.

Delnevo CD, Abatemarco DJ, Steinberg MB. Physician response rates to a mail survey by specialty and timing of incentive. *American Journal of Preventive Medicine* 2004; 26(3): 234–236.

Demirsoy N, Kirimlioglu N. Protection of privacy and confidentiality as a patient right: physicians' and nurses' viewpoints. *Biomedical Research* 2016; 27(4).

Dharamsi S, Ho A, Spadafora SM et al. The physician as health advocate: translating the quest for social responsibility into medical education and practice. *Academic Medicine* 2011; 86(9): 1108–1113.

Dictionnaire de l'Académie française, 9e éd. Disponible: <https://www.dictionnaire-academie.fr/article/A9R209>.

Division de la population de l'ONU: Perspectives de la population mondiale: Révision de 2015. New York: United nations; 2015. Disponible: <http://esa.un.org/unpd/wpp/>

Division de la population de l'ONU: World urbanization prospects: the 2014 revision. New York: United nations; 2014. Disponible: <https://www.un.org/en/development/desa/publications/2014-revision-world-urbanization-prospects.html>

Drysdale A, Blake GH. *The Middle East and North Africa*. USA: Oxford University Press; 1985.

Duggirala M. Patient-perceived dimensions of total quality service in healthcare. *Benchmarking An International Journal* 2008; 15(5): 560–583.

Duong Quynh Lien, La responsabilité sociale de l'entreprise, pourquoi et comment ça se parle? . *Communication et organisation* 2005; 26: 26–43.

Durán A, Kutzin J, Martin-Moreno JM et al. Understanding health systems: scope, functions and objectives. In: *Health systems: Health, wealth, society and wellbeing*. Maidenhead: NY Open University Press, McGraw Hill; 2011, pp. 19–37.

Eckardt KU et al. Evolving importance of kidney disease: from subspecialty to global health burden. *Lancet* 2013; 382: 158–69.

Education in Africa. UNESCO Institute of Statistics; 2020.

Ekpe EE, Ekirikpo U. Challenges of vascular access in a new dialysis centre – Uyo experience. *Pan African Medical* 2010; 7: 23.

Eleanor Lederer. Women in nephrology today. *Clinical Journal of the American Society of Nephrology* 2018; 13: 1755–1756.

Esposito P, Dal Canton A. Clinical audit, a valuable tool to improve quality of care: general methodology and applications in nephrology. *World Journal of Nephrology* 2014; 3(4): 249–255

Essoungou AM. La bonne gouvernance, clé du progrès. *Afrique Renouveau*; août 2010.

Essue BM, Laba M, Knaul F et al. Economic burden of chronic ill health and injuries for households in low- and middle-income countries. In: Jamison DT, Gelband H, Horton S, et al., eds. *Disease control priorities: improving health and reducing poverty*. 3rd ed. Washington, DC: The International Bank for Reconstruction and Development / The World Bank; 2017.

État de la santé dans la région africaine de l'OMS: analyse de la situation sanitaire, des services et des systèmes de santé dans le contexte des objectifs de développement durable. Organisation mondiale de la Santé, Bureau régional de l'Afrique; 2018.

European Union Sex ratio. Index mundi, CIA World Factbook; 2018. Disponible: <https://www.indexmundi.com/european_union/sex_ratio.html>

Fadare JO, Adeoti AO, Desalu OO et al. The prescribing of generic medicines in Nigeria: knowledge, perceptions and attitudes of physicians. *Expert Review of Pharmacoeconomics & Outcomes Research* 2016; 16(5): 639–650.

Fan W, Yen Z. Factors affecting response rates of the web survey: a systematic review. *Computers in Human Behavior* 2009; 26(2): 132–139.

Feehally J, Brusselmans A, Finkelstein FO et al. Improving global health: measuring the success of capacity building outreach programs: a view from the International Society of Nephrology. *Kidney International* 2016; 6: 42–51.

Fenton JJ; Jerant AF; Bertakis KD. The cost of satisfaction: a national study of patient satisfaction, health care utilization, expenditures, and mortality. *Archives of Internal Medicine* 2012; 172(5): 405–11.

Fokou M, Ashuntantang G, Teyang A et al. Patients characteristics and outcome of 518 arterioveinous fistulas for hemodialysis in Sub-Saharian African setting. *Annals of Vascular Surgery* 2012; 26: 674–679.

Fottler MD, Blair JD. *Challenges in health care management strategic perspectives for managing key stakeholders*. Jossey-Bass. 1990.

Francis CK. The medical ethos and social responsibility in clinical medicine. *Journal of the National Medical Association* 2001; 93: 157–169.

Freeman RE. *Strategic management: a stakeholder approach*. Boston: Pitman; 1984.

Friedberg MW, Chen PG, Van Busum KR et al. Factors affecting physician professional satisfaction and their implications for patient care, health systems, and health policy. *RAND Health Quarterly* 2014; 3(4): 1.

Friedericksen DV, Van der Merwe L, Hattingh TL et al. Acute renal failure in the medical ICU still predictive of high mortality. *South African Medical Journal* 2009; 99: 873–875.

Frunză S. Ethical responsibility and social responsibility of organizations involved in the public health system. *Revista de cercetare și intervenție socială* 2011; 32: 155–171.

Garcia-Garcia G, Garcia-Bejarano H, Breien-Coronado H et al. End-stage renal disease in Mexico. In: Garcia-Garcia G, Agodoa L, Norris K, eds. *Chronic kidney disease in disadvantaged populations*. New York, NY: Elsevier; 2017: 77–82.

Gething PW, Noor AM, Gikandi PW et al. Improving imperfect data from health management information systems in Africa using space-time geostatistics. *PLoS Med* 2006; 3: e271.

Ghose A, Adhsih VS. Patient satisfaction with medical services: hospital-based study. *Health and Population* 2011; 34(4): 232–242.

Global consensus on social accountability of medical schools. GCSA conference; Oct. 10–13, 2010; East London, South Africa; 2010 Disponible: <www.healthsocialaccountability.org>.

Global strategy on human resources for health: workforce 2030. WHO; 2016.

Godman B, Abuelkhair M, Vitry A et al. Payers endorse generics to enhance prescribing efficiency; impact and future implications, a case history approach. *GaBI* 2012; 1(2): 21–35.

Gond JP, Igalens J. La responsabilité sociale de l'entreprise. Que sais-je? 5e éd. France: PUF; 2016.

Görgen H, Kirsch-Woik T, Schmidt-Ehry R. Le Système de santé de district. Expériences et perspectives en Afrique. Manuel à l'intention des professionnels de santé publique. 2e éd. Wersbaden: GTZ; 2004.

Graham H. Social determinants and their unequal distribution: clarifying policy understandings. *Milbank Quarterly* 2004; 82: 101–124.

Guinée: la pêche industrielle interdite pendant deux mois [archive]. RFI; 2 juill. 2016.

Guttmann A, Schull MJ, Vermeulen MJ et al. Association between waiting times and short term mortality and hospital admission after departure from emergency department: population based cohort study from Ontario, Canada. *BMJ* 2011; 342: d2983.

Haddiya I. Focus sur la transplantation rénale. *Revue de médecine générale et de famille* 2010; 10: 86–92.

Halle MP, Nyongbella J, Fouda H et al. Factors associated with late presentation of patients with chronic kidney disease in nephrology consultation in Cameroon-a descriptive cross-sectional study. *Renal Failure* 2019; 41(1): 384–392.

Halle MPE, Kengne AP, Ashuntantang G. Referral of patients with kidney impairment for specialist care in a developing country of Sub-Saharan Africa. *Renal Failure* 2009; 31: 341–348.

Hamel K, Tong, Hofer M. Poverty in Africa is now falling – but not fast enough. Brookings 2019.

Hammach M. L'impact de la responsabilité sociale de l'entreprise sur l'implication organisationnelle des cadres salariés: cas du secteur de l'industrie agroalimentaire au Maroc. Gestion et management. Conservatoire national des arts et metiers – CNAM, 2016. NNT: 2016CNAM1092.

Harris DCH, Dupuis S, Couser WG et al. Training nephrologists from developing countries: does it have a positive impact? *Kidney International* 2012; Suppl. 2: 275–278.

Heald M. The social responsabilities of business. Company and community, 1900–1960. Cleveland: Press of case western Reserve University; 1970; Pasquero J. La responsabilité sociale de l'entreprise comme objet des sciences de gestion: un regard historique » in M.-F. Bouthillier- Turcotte, A. Salmon, Responsabilité sociale et environnementale de l'entreprise, Sillery, Presses de l'Université du Québec; 2005, pp. 80–112.

Health system strategy. WHO; 2007. Disponible: <http://www.who.int/health systems/strategy/en/>

Health systems in Africa- Community perceptions and perspectives. The report of a multi-country study. World Health Organization, Regional office for Africa: 2012.

Hugon P. L'Afrique: Défis, enjeux et perspectives en 40 fiches pour comprendre l'actualité. Eyrolles éditions; 2016. Disponible: <https://www.eyrolles.com/Chapitres/9782212564846/9782212564846.pdf>

Hwang HS et al. Comparison of clinical outcome between twice-weekly and thrice-weekly hemodialysis in patients with residual kidney function. *Medicine* (Baltimore) 2016; 95: e2767.

Integrating Population Issues into Sustainable Development, including the post-2015 Development Agenda: a concise report: publication des Nations Unies. United nations; 2015. Disponible: <www.un.org/en/development/desa/population/commission/pdf/48/CPD48ConciseReport.pdf>.

Investir dans la santé en Afrique. Harmonisation pour la santé en Afrique. OMS; 2011. Disponible: <https://www.who.int/pmnch/media/membernews/2011/investir_sante_afrique.pdf?ua=1>.

Investir dans la santé en Afrique. Le secteur privé: un partenaire pour améliorer les conditions de vie des populations. Washington: Groupe de la Banque mondiale; 2008.

Islam F, Rahman A, Halim A et al. Perceptions of health care providers and patients on quality of care in maternal and neonatal health in fourteen Bangladesh government healthcare facilities: a mixed-method study. *BMC Health Services Research* 2015; 15 : 237.

Islam MM. Social determinants of health and related inequalities: confusion and implications. *Frontiers in Public Health* 2019; 7:11.

Jacquemot P. Les classes moyennes changent-elles la donne en Afrique? Réalités, enjeux et perspectives. *Afrique contemporaine* 2012; 244: 17–31

Jacquemot P. Les systèmes de santé en Afrique et l'inégalité face aux soins. *Afrique contemporaine* 2012: 3(243); 95–97.

Kakabadse N, Rozuel C. Meaning of corporate social responsibility in a local French hospital: a case study. *Society and Business Review* 2006; 1: 77–96.

Kane Y, Cisse MM, Gaye M, et al. Problematic of vascular access for hemodialysis in sub-Saherienne Africa: Experience of Dakar. *Journal of Nephrology & Therapeutics* 2015; 5: 216.

Kashyap R et al. Corporate social responsibility: a call for multidisciplinary inquiry. *Journal of Business & Economics Research* 2004; 2(7): 51–58.

Keyvanara M, Sajadi HS. Social responsibility of the hospitals in Isfahan city, Iran: results from a cross-sectional survey. *International Journal of Health Policy and Management* 2015; 4(8): 517–522.

Kidney Disease: Improving Global Outcomes (KDIGO) CKD Work Group. KDIGO 2012 clinical practice guideline for the evaluation and management of chronic kidney disease. *Kidney International* 2013; (suppl 3): 1–150.

Kirigia JM, Barry SP. Health challenges in Africa and the way forward. *International Archives of Medicine* 2008, 1: 27.

Knapp van Bogaert D. Ethics CPD supplement: ethics in health care: confidentiality and information technologies. *South African Family Practice* 2014; 56(1) (Suppl 1): S3–S5.

Kotzian P. Determinants of satisfaction with health care system. *Open Political Science Journal* 2009; 2(1): 47–58.

Kuikeu O. Conséquences de l'instabilité politique de l'Afrique: la trappe de la dépendance à l'égard des matières premières » [archive]. Atelier des médias, RFI, 12 juill. 2012.

Kurniawan R. Effect of environmental performance on environmental disclosures of manufacturing, mining and plantation companies listed in Indonesia stock exchange. *Arthatama: Journal of Business Management and Accounting* 2017; 1 (1): 6–17.

Kurt Darr. The social responsability of hospitals. *Hospital Topics* 1997; 75(1).

La banque mondiale: Indicateurs 2020. Banque mondiale; 2020. Disponible: <https://donnees.banquemondiale.org/indicateur>.

La dialyse péritonéale et les autres techniques. RDPLF; 2012. Disponible: <https://www.rdplf.org/279-liens-gene-autres-techniques.html>.

La diversification économique: une urgence pour l'Afrique. Afrique renouveau. Nations unies; avr. 2011. p. 26.

La Rosa E et al. Social responsibility in health and the global health situation: towards new health and social indicators. *Revue de santé publique* 2007; 19(3): 217–227.

La Rosa E, Dubois G, Tonnellier F. Social responsibility in health and the global health situation: towards new health and social indicators. *Revue de santé publique* 2007; 19(3): 217–227.

Lacson E Jr., Wang W, Lazarus JM et al. Hemodialysis facility-based quality-of-care indicators and facility-specific patient outcomes. *American Journal of Kidney Diseases* 2009; 54: 490–497.

Lavy V, Strauss J, Duncan Thomas et al. Quality of health care, survival and health outcomes in Ghana *Journal of Health Economics* 1996; 15: 333–357.

Lee M, Kohler J. Benchmarking and transparency: incentives for the pharmaceutical industry's corporate social responsibility. *Journal of Business Ethics* 2010; 95(4): 641–658.

Legendre C. La transplantation rénale. Paris: Médecine sciences publications Lavoisier; 2012.

Leisinger KM. The corporate social responsibility of the pharmaceutical industry: idealism without illusion and realism without resignation. *Business Ethics Quarterly* 2005; 15(4): 577–594.

Levitt T. The dangers of social responsibility. *Harvard Business Review* 1958; 36: 41–50.

Lin YF et al. Comparison of residual renal function in patients undergoing twice-weekly versus three-times-weekly haemodialysis. *Nephrology* 2009; 14: 59–64.

Liu W, Shi L, Pong RW et al. How patients think about social responsibility of public hospitals in China?. *BMC Health Services Research* 2016; 16: 371.

Loi n° 16-98 relative au don, au prélèvement et à la transplantation d'organes et de tissus humains. *Bulletin officiel* n: 5480– 15 Kaada 1427 (7-12-2006).

Lopera-Medina MM. Utilización de servicios de salud por enfermedades catastró cas o de alto costo en Antioquia. *Rev Gerenc Polít Salud* 2017; 16(32): 120–137.

Lubis AN. Corporate social responsibility in health sector: a case study in the government hospitals in Medan, Indonesia. Verslas: Teorija Ir Praktika / Business: Theory and practice. 2018; 19: 25–36.

Lucyk K, McLaren L. Taking stock of the social determinants of health: a scoping review. *PLoS ONE* 2017; 12(5): e0177306.

Lumenganeso O. L'Afrique doit d'abord investir dans ses infrastructures. *Les Afriques*; 31 août 2010.

Luyckx VA et al. Equity and economics of kidney disease in sub-Saharan Africa. *Lancet* 2013; 382: 103–104.

Magill G, Prybil L. Stewardship and integrity in health care: a role for organizational ethics. *Journal of Business Ethics* 2004; 50(3): 225–238.

Martinez-Palomo A. The UNESCO Universal Declaration on Bioethics and Human Rights.

Martinez-Palomo A. The UNESCO Universal Declaration on Bioethics and Human Rights. Background, principles and application Paris: UNESCO Publishing; 2009.

Mathebeni-Bokwe P. Management of medical records for healthcare service delivery at the Victoria Public Hospital in the Eastern Cape Province: South Africa (thesis). Alice (South Africa): Fort Hare Univ.; 2015. Disponible: <https://pdfs.semanticscholar.org/e888/2023a43f5266449c6eed35f092f02e47163f.pdf>.

Mathebeni-Bokwe P. Management of medical records for healthcare service delivery at the Victoria Public Hospital in the Eastern Cape Province: South Africa (thesis). Alice (South Africa): Fort Hare Univ.; 2015. Disponible: <https://pdfs.semanticscholar.org/e888/2023a43f5266449c6eed35f092f02e47163f.pdf>.

Matignon M et al. Transplantation rénale: indications, résultats, limites et perspectives. *La Presse médicale* 2007; 36: 1829–1834.

McGraw D, Greene SM, Miner CS et al. Privacy and confidentiality in pragmatic clinical trials. *Clinical Trials* 2015; 12(5): 520–529.

Meili R, Buchman S. La responsabilité sociale: au cœur de la médecine familiale. *Canadian Family Physician* 2013; 59(4): 344–345.

Mercandalli S, Losch B. Rural Africa in motion. Dynamics and drivers of migration South of the Sahara. Rome: FAO and CIRAD; 2017.

Meyer JA, Silow-Carroll S, Stepnick LS et al. Hospital quality: ingredients for success – overview and lessons learned. New York, NY: The Commonwealth Fund; 2004.

Mitra S, Posarac A, Vick B. "Disability and poverty in developing countries: a snapshot from the World Health Survey". Social protection and labor. Washington, DC: The World Bank. 2011; pp. 33–34.

Monitoring the building blocks of health systems: a handbook of indicators and their measurement strategies. Disponible: <http://www.who.int/healthinfo/systems/monitoring/en/>.

Monot T, Afrique (Structure et milieu). Biogéographie, Encyclopædia Universalis. Éditeur Primento; 2016.

Moosa MR, Kidd M. The dangers of rationing dialysis treatment: the dilemma facing a developing country. *Kidney International* 2006; 70: 1107–1114.

Morton RL, Tong A, Howard K et al. The views of patients and carers in treatment decision making for chronic kidney disease: systematic review and thematic synthesis of qualitative studies. *BMJ* 2010; 340: c112.

Mullan F, Frehywot S, Omaswa F et al. Medical schools in sub-Saharan Africa. *Lancet* 2011; 377: 1113–1121.

Muller E, Barday Z, Mendelson M et al. Renal transplantation between HIV-positive donors and recipients justified. *South African Medical Journal* 2012; 102: 497–498.

Muller E. Transplantation in Africa. *Clinical Nephrology* 2016; 86: Suppl. 1 (90 – 95).

Mungai C. Sex ratios In Africa: where women outnumber men, and vice versa, and why it matters. *Africa pedia*; 2017. Disponible: <https://africapedia.com/sex-ratio-africa/>

Musau Z. Africa grapples with huge disparities in education. Africa renewal; 2018.

Naicker S. End-stage renal disease in sub-Saharan Africa. *Ethnicity & Disease* 2009; 19: S1–13–5.

Naidu A. Factors affecting patient satisfaction and healthcare quality. *International Journal of Health Care Quality Assurance* 2009; 22(4): 366–381.

Netter FH. *Atlas d'anatomie humaine*. 6e éd. France: Elsevier Masson; 2015.

Ngoepe M. An exploration of records management trends in the South African public sector. *Mousaion* 2009; 27: 116–136.

Nguyen Thi PL, Frimat L, Loos-Ayav C. SDIALOR: a dialysis patient satisfaction questionnaire. *Néphrologie & Thérapeutique* 2008; 4: 266–277.

Nirupam M. Attitudes and perceptions of medical doctors towards their jobs in the state of J&K, *India International Journal of Health* 2007; 1, No.2.

Nwankwo EA, Wudiri WW, Bassi A. Practice pattern of hemodialysis vascular access in Maiduguri, Nigeria. *The International Journal of Artificial Organs* 2006; 29: 956e60.

Nylenna M, Riis P. Identification of patients in medical publications: need for informed consent. *British Medical Journal* 1991; 302:1182.

Observatoire mondial de la santé de l'OMS. OMS; 2020.

Observatoire mondial de la santé de l'OMS. OMS; 2020. Disponible: <https://www.who.int/gho/database/fr/>

Observatoire mondial de la santé de l'OMS. OMS; 2020. Disponible: <https://www.who.int/gho/database/fr/>

Oger C. *Corporate social responsibility in the pharmaceutical industry: between trend and necessity*. Library and Archives Canada; 2010.

Okel J, Okpechi IG, Qarni B et al. Nephrology training curriculum and implications for optimal kidney care in the developing world. *Clinical Nephrology* 2016; 86: 110–113.

Okpechi I, Rayner BL, Swanepoel C. Peritoneal dialysis in Cape Town, South Africa. *Peritoneal Dialysis International* 2012; 32: 254–260.

Okunola OO, Ayodele OE, Adekanle AD. Acute kidney injury requiring hemodialysis in the tropics. *Saudi Journal of Kidney Diseases and Transplantation* 2012; 23: 1315–1319.

OMS, UNICEF, FNUAP, Groupe de la Banque mondiale et Division de la population des Nations Unies, Tendances de la mortalité maternelle: 1990–2015. Genève: Organisation mondiale de la santé; 2015. Disponible à l'adresse: <http://apps.who.int/iris/bitstream/10665/194254/1/9789241565141_eng.pdf>.

Ormandy P. Information topics important to chronic kidney disease patients: a systematic review. *Journal of Renal Care* 2008; 34: 19–27.

Ortiz-Prado E, Fors M, Henriquez-Trujillo. AR et al. Attitudes and perceptions of medical doctors towards the local health system: a questionnaire survey in Ecuador. *BMC Health Services Research* 2019; 19: 363.

Ortiz-Prado E, Ponce J, Cornejo-Leon F et al. Analysis of health and drug access associated with the purchasing power of the Ecuadorian population. *Global Journal of Health Science* 2017; 9(1): 201–210.

Osborn R, Squires D, Doty MM et al. In New Survey of Eleven Countries, US adults still struggle with access to and affordability of health care. *Health Affairs* 2016; 35(12): 2327–2336.

Osman MA et al. Health workforce for nephrology care: existing manpower and training capacity. *Kidney International Supplements* 2018; 8: 52–63.

Pak Sum Low. *Climate change and Africa*. Cambridge University Press; 2006.

Palmer SC, de Berardis G, Craig JC et al. Patient satisfaction with in-centre haemodialysis care: an international survey. *BMJ Open* 2014; 4: e005020.

Parker MG, Pivert KA, Ibrahim T, Molitoris recruiting the next generation of nephrologists. *Advances in Chronic Kidney Disease* 2013 July; 20(4): 326–335.

Perspectives économiques en Afrique – Gouvernance politique et économique en Afrique. 2016; 5: 131.

Perspectives économiques en Afrique 2011. OECD, African Development Bank, United Nations Economic Commission for Africa. United Nations Development Programme; 2011

Perspectives économiques en Afrique 2019. Groupe de la banque africaine de développement; 2019

Peters DH, Garg A, Bloom G et al. Poverty and access to health care in developing countries. *Annals of the New York Academy of Sciences* 2008; 1136(1): 161–171.

Pinheiro J. The physician-patient relationship in dialysis. *Portuguese Journal of Nephrology and Hypertension* 2013; 27(3): 179–185.

Pitte JR. Atlas de l'Afrique, Les éditions du Jaguar; 2011.

Polle B. Afrique de l'Ouest: les rouages de la pêche illégale passés au crible. *Jeune Afrique* 29 jui. 2016.

Poor health systems and lack of infrastructure paralyses health care in Africa. AFRIC Editorial; Dec. 2018. Disponible: <https://afric.online/5626-poor-health-systems-and-lack-of-infrastructure-paralyses-health-care-in-africa/>.

Population Finder. United States Census Bureau; 2008. Disponible: from:<http://factfinder.census.gov/servlet/SAFFPopulation?_sse=on>

Powers M et Faden R. *Social justice: the moral foundations of public health and health policy* (Issues in Biomedical ethics). New York: Oxford University Press; 2006.

Prakash S, O'Hare AM. Interaction of aging and CKD. *Seminars in Nephrology* 2009; 29(5): 497–503.

Pras B, Evrard Y, Roux E, Market: études et recherches en marketing – Fondements, méthodes. 3e éd: Dunod; 2003 p. 704.

Profil démographique de l'Afrique. Addis-Abeba (Éthiopie): Commission économique des Nations Unies pour l'Afrique; Mar. 2018. Groupe de la publication et de l'impression de la CEA, certifié ISO 14001:2004.

Profil démographique de l'Afrique. Addis-Abeba (Éthiopie): Commission -

Pulley Sayre A. Africa. Twenty-First Century Books; 1999.

Questions and Answers on Universal Health Coverage. World Health Organization; 2020. Disponible: <https://www.who.int/healthsystems/topics/financing/uhc_qa/en/>.

Ramdani B et al. Consideration on the implementation of a registry of renal transplant recipients and a registry of living donors in the Maghreb countries. *Nephrology & Therapeutics* 2015; 11(6): 521–524.

Rapport du Comité international de bioéthique de l'UNESCO (CIB) sur LA RESPONSABILITÉ SOCIALE ET LA SANTÉ, Publié par l'Organisation des Nations Unies pour l'éducation, la science et la culture. UNESCO 2010.

Rapport enquête satisfaction patients dialysés. AURAL; 2014.

Rapport sur la compétitivité en Afrique 2015: Transformer les économies africaines [archive]. Banque mondiale; 2015.

Rapport sur la santé dans le monde, 2000 – Pour un système de santé plus performant, Genève: Organisation mondiale de la Santé; 2000. Disponible: <http://www.who.int/iris/handle/10665/42281>

Recommandations de bonnes pratiques médicales. ALD 17: Insuffisance rénale terminale. SMN; 2013.

Renforcement des systèmes de santé: Quelles perspectives pour les initiatives mondiales pour la santé? WHO; 2006. Disponible: <https://www.who.int/management/working_paper_4_fr_opt.pdf>.

Report: Income Inequality Skewed Wealth, Resources to Pockets of 20% of Nigerians. This Day Business Newspaper June 2016.

Revicki DA. Gut 2004; 53(Suppl IV): iv40–iv44.

Revision of World Population Prospects. World Economic Forum. United Nations; 2019.

Richardson MM, Paine SS, Grobert ME, Satisfaction with Care of Patients on Hemodialysis. *Clinical Journal of the American Society of Nephrology* 2015; 10(8): 1428–1434.

Riman HB, Akpan ES. Healthcare financing and health outcomes in Nigeria: a state level study using multivariate analysis. *International Journal of Humanities and Social Science* 2012; 15: 296–309.

Rohini R, Mahadevappa B. Social responsibility of hospitals: an Indian context. Social Responsibility Journal 2010; 6 (2): 268–285.

Rosoff PM. Can the case report withstand ethical scrutiny? *Hastings Center Report* 2019; 49(6): 17–21.

Ross CK, Steward CA, Sinacore JM. A comparative study of seven measures of patient satisfaction. Medical Care 1995; 33: 392–406.

Rotenstein LS, Huckman RS, Wagle NW. Making patients and doctors happier – the potential of patient-reported outcomes. *The New England Journal of Medicine* 2017; 377: 1309–1312.

Rural Development Report Creating opportunities for rural youth. Rome: IFAD (International Fund for Agricultural Development); 2019.

Sainsaulieu R. *Lentreprise, une affaire de société*. Paris: Presses de sciences Po; 1992.

Salsberg E, Masselink L, Wu X. *The US nephrology workforce: Developments and trends*. Washington, DC: American Society of Nephrology; 2014.

Sankar P, Mora S, Merz J et al. Patient perspectives of medical confidentiality: a review of the literature. *Journal of General Internal Medicine* 2003; 18: 659–669.

Satoshi I, Tetsuji K, Yasuo O et al. Analysis of 2897 hospitalization events for patients with chronic kidney disease: results from CKD-JAC study. *Clinical and Experimental Nephrology* 2019; (23): 956–968.

Savla D, Chertow GM, Meyer T et al. Can twice weekly hemodialysis expand patient access under resource constraints? *Hemodialysis International* 2017; 21(4): 445–452.

Schermerhorn JR. *Management*. 6th Asia-Pacific ed. Melbourne: Wiley; 2016.

Sex Ratio in Africa. African development Bank Group; Aug. 2019. Disponible sur: <https://dataportal.opendataforafrica.org/ouhoojg/sex-ratio-in-africa>

Shaping Corporate Social Responsibility in sub-Saharan Africa Guidance. Notes from a Mapping Survey. GIZ Center for Cooperation with Private Sector and University of Stellenbosch; 2013. Disponible: <https://www.giz.de/expertise/downloads/giz2013-en-africa-csr-mapping.pdf>

Singh K, Diamantidis CJ, Ramani S et al. Patients' and nephrologists' evaluation of patient-facing smartphone apps for CKD. *Clinical Journal of the American Society of Nephrology* 2019; 14: 523–529.

Siniora D. *Corporate social responsibility in the health care sector. 4th annual student symposium.* Dusquene Univ. Dusquene Scholarship collection; Aug. 25th. 2017.

Solberg B, Tómasson K, Aasland O et al. Cross-national comparison of job satisfaction in doctors during economic recession. *Occupational Medicine* 2014; 64(8): 595–600.

Soors et al. Lack of access to health care for African indigents: a social exclusion perspective. *International Journal for Equity in Health* 2013, 12: 91.

Spencer E et al. *Organization ethics in health care.* Oxford: Oxford University Press; 2000.

Squires D, Anderson C. US health care from a global perspective: spending, use of services, prices, and health in 13 countries. Commonwealth Fund 2015; 15: 1–16.

Stanifer JW et al. The epidemiology of chronic kidney disease in sub-Saharan Africa: a systematic review and meta-analysis. *The Lancet. Global Health* 2014; 2(3): e174–e181.

Statistiques sanitaires mondiales 2017: Suivi de la santé pour les ODD. Organisation mondiale de la santé; 2017.

Steinman TI. Nephrology workforce shortfall: solutions are needed. *American Journal of Kidney Diseases* 1999; 33: 798–800.

Stenberg K, Hanssen O, Edejer TT et al. Financing transformative health systems towards achievement of the health Sustainable Development Goals: a model for projected resource needs in 67 low-income and middle-income countries. *The Lancet. Global Health* 2017; 5: e875–e877.

Stiglitz J. *Globalization and its discontents.* Fayard: Paris; 2002.

Strasser R, Kam SM, Regalado SM. Rural health care access and policy in developing countries. *Annual Review of Public Health* 2016; 37: 395–412.

Strengthening health systems to improve health outcomes: WHO's framework for action. Geneva: WHO; 2007.

Sud N. *Health and education in Africa*. World Bank group; 2020. Disponible: <https://www.ifc.org/wps/wcm/connect/REGION__EXT_Content/Regions/Sub-Saharan+Africa/Investments/HealthEducation/>.

Suliman AA, Eltom M, Elmadhoun WM. Factors affecting job satisfaction among junior doctors working at teaching hospitals in River Nile State, Sudan. *Journal of Public Health and Emergency* 2017; 1: 79.

Swanepoel CR, Wearne N, Okpechi IG. Nephrology in Africa – not yet uhuru. *Nature Reviews Nephrology* 2013 Oct.; 9(10): 610–622.

Swanson RC et al. Toward a consensus on guiding principles for health systems strengthening. *PLoS Med* 2010; 7(12): e1000385.

t Hoen EF, Hogerzeil HV, Quick JD. A quiet revolution in global public health: the World Health Organization's prequalification of medicines programme. *Journal of Public Health Policy* 2014; 35(2): 137–161.

Tadese T, Mohamed A, Mengistie A. Assessment of factors influencing job satisfaction among health care providers, federal police referral hospital, Addis Ababa, Ethiopia. *Ethiopian Journal of Health Development* 2015; 29: 119–126.

Takahashi T et al. Corporate social responsibility and hospitals: US theory, Japanese experiences, and lessons for other countries. *Healthcare Management* 2013; 26(4): 176–179.

Task shifting to tackle health worker shortages – global recommendations and guidelines. WHO; 2008. Disponible: <http://www.who.int/healthsystems/task_shifting/en/>.

The 2007 Global Business Barometer. Economist Intelligence Unit. The Economist 2008.

The middle class in Africa realities and challenges. CFAO; 2015. Disponible: <http://www.cfaogroup.com/static/2017/12/08/CFAO-White%20Paper%20The%20middle%20classes%20in%20Africa%20UK%20april2016.pdf?qA3g3_m5sGX6zBNHJgp4PQ:qA3g3_m5sGX6zBNHJgp4PQ:fIcrNtDaj1kHsdVnXP2w9g>.

Topf JM, Hiremath S. Got CKD? There's an app for that! *Clinical Journal of the American Society of Nephrology* 2019; 14: 491–492.

Tout l'univers- Encyclopédie. *Le livre de Paris-Hachette*. Paris: Hachette Collections SNC; 2014.

Townsend BA. Privacy and Data protection ehealth in Africa (PhD thesis). South Africa: Univ. of Cape Town; 2017.

Tyssen R, Palmer KS, Solberg IB. Physicians' perceptions of quality of care, professional autonomy, and job satisfaction in Canada, Norway, and the United States. *BMC Health Services Research* 2013; 13: 516.

U.S. Renal Data System. USRDS 2012 Annual Data Report: Atlas of Chronic Kidney Disease and End-Stage Renal Disease in the United States. Bethesda: National Institutes of Health, National Institute of Diabetes and Digestive and Kidney Diseases; 2012.

Universal Health coverage. Regional office for Africa. WHO; 2019.

Van Biesen W, Jha V, Abu-Alfa AK. Considerations on equity in management of end-stage kidney disease in low- and middle-income countries. *Kidney International Supplements* 2020; 10: e63–e71.

Van Hoving DJ, Brysiewicz P. African emergency care providers' attitudes and practices towards research. *African Journal of Emergency Medicine* 2017; 7: 9e14.

Van Lerberghe W, De Brouwere V. État de santé et santé de l'État en Afrique subsaharienne. *Afrique contemporaine* 2000; 195: 175–190.

Wachterman M, Marcantonio E, Davis R et al. Relationship between the prognostic expectations of seriously ill patients undergoing hemodialysis and their nephrologists. *JAMA Internal Medicine* 2013; 173: 1206–1214.

Waddock S. The difference makers. How social and institutional entrepreneurs created the Corporate Responsibility Movement. Sheffield: Greenleaf Publishing; 2008.

Walker RJ, Smalls BL, Campbell JA et al. Impact of social determinants of health on outcomes for type 2 diabetes: a systematic review. *Endocrine* 2014 Sept; 47(1): 29–48.

Weaver M, Patrick DL, Markson LE et al. Issues in the measurement of satisfaction with treatment. *American Journal of Managed Care* 1997; 3: 579–594.

Whitworth JA, Kokwaro G, Kinyanjui S et al. Strengthening capacity for health research in Africa. *Lancet* 2008; 372: 1590e3.

Will T, Saudan P, Droulez MG et al. Relationship and dependency in a hemodialysis unit. *Néphrologie et thérapeutique* 2008; 4: 320–324.

Wong REX, Bradley EH. Developing patient registration and medical records management system in Ethiopia. *International Journal for Quality in Health Care* 2009; 21(4): 253–258.

Wood DJ. Corporate Social Performance revisited. Academy of Management Review 1991; 16(4): 691–718; Frederick WC, From CSR1 to CRS2: the maturing of business and society thought. Working paper graduate school of business. Pittsburgh, PA: Pittsburgh Univ.; 1978.

Wood DJ. Corporate Social Performance revisited. *Academy of Management Review* 1991; 16(4): 691–718.

World Bank staff estimates based on the United Nations Population Division's World Urbanization Prospects. World bank; 2018.

World development indicators. World Bank; 2020. Disponible: <http://data.worldbank.org/indicator/SH>. XPD. PC AP.

Wu CC. The impact of hospital brand image on service quality, patient satisfaction and loyalty. *African Journal of Business Management* 2011; 5(12): 4873.

Wunch G et al. Socioeconomic differences in mortality: a life course approach. *European Journal of Population* 1996; 12: 167–185.

Xesfingi S, Vozikis A. Patient satisfaction with the healthcare system: assessing the impact of socio-economic and healthcare provision factors. *BMC Health Services Research* 2016; 16: 94.

Yahia M. *Africa's defining challenge*. Africa: UNDP; 2017.

Table of contents

Abbreviations 15

Introduction 17

Part I: Social responsibility in healthcare

Chapter 1: Corporate social responsibility 23
    I. The concept of responsibility 23
        1. What is responsibility? 23
        2. The different types of responsibility 23
    II. Corporate social responsibility (CSR) 24
        1. Corporate social responsibility 24
        2. The foundations of CSR 25
        3. CSR: Advocates vs. opponents 26
        4. The institutionalisation and theoretical foundations of CSR 27
        5. CSR: A theory of stakeholders 28
        6. Measuring CSR 29
        7. The financial impact of CSR 30
        8. CSR economic and managerial implications 30
    III. Health-focussed corporate social responsibility (CSR) 31
        1. CSR: Health investments 31
        2. CSR approaches to healthcare 32
    IV. Corporate social responsibility in healthcare 33
        1. Social responsibility in healthcare: The role of health care organisations and pharmaceutical industries 34
        2. Social responsibility and health governance 35
        3. Social responsibility in healthcare: The role of health care managers and leaders 35

Chapter 2: The values and obligations of health care organisations 37
    1. The values of social responsibility in healthcare 37
    2. The ethics of healthcare organisations 38
    3. Social responsibility in healthcare: A moral obligation 40

Chapter 3: The ethical principles of social responsibility in healthcare 43
    1. The principle of justice 43
    2. The principle of beneficence 43

Chapter 4: Social responsibility of faculties of medicine 45
    1. Social responsibility in healthcare: The role of faculties of medicine 45

Chapter 5: The social determinants of health 47
    1. What are the social determinants of health? 47
    2. The social determinants of health: An ambiguous concept ... 49
    3. Actions related to the social determinants of health 49

Part II: The situation of health in Africa

Chapter 1: The context and situation of health in Africa 53
    I. The African continent: 53
        1.1. African demographics 55
        1.2. African society 59
        1.3. African economy 59
    II. The situation of health in Africa 63
    III. The health situation of African populations 64
    IV. Healthcare systems in Africa 69
    V. The performance of healthcare systems in Africa 72
    VI. The situation of investments in healthcare systems 74
        *The sources of health financing 77

    *The management of health funds 77
    *Service procurement 77
    *Health information systems (HIS) 78
    *Health surveys and census 78
    *Health research 79

Chapter 2: African nephrology 81
    1. What is nephrology? 81
    2. The kidney: A multifunctional organ 81
    3. Chronic kidney disease 82
    4. Acute kidney failure 83
    5. What is kidney replacement therapy (KRT)? 83
     *When to consider the replacement therapy? 83
     * The informed choice of the replacement therapy 84
     * Hemodialysis 84
     *Peritoneal dialysis 85
     *Kidney transplantation 86
    6. Nephrology in Africa 87
    7. Kidney disease in Africa: Epidemiological data 88
     *Hemodialysis 92
     *Peritoneal dialysis (PD) 93
     *Kidney transplantation in Africa 94

Part III: Social responsibility in healthcare: An African-wide survey

Chapter 1: An African-wide survey 99

Chapter 2: Patients: The characteristics and perceptions of hospital social responsibility 101
    1. The targeted patients: Recruitment challenges 101

2. The socio-economic characteristics of the targeted countries	103
3. The provision of nephrology care by country	104
4. Patient demographics	105
5. Patients' socio-economic data	108
6. Patients' renal data	114
7. Patients' perceptions of hospital social responsibility	120

Chapter 3: Nephrologists: The characteristics and perceptions of hospital social responsibility 143

    *Quality of care   148
    *Access to health care   152
    *Professional ethics   157

Chapter 4: Factors influencing hospital social responsibility 169

    1. Patient-related factors: 169
    2. Doctor-related factors 170
    3. Hospital-related factors 172
    4. Health system-related factors 173

Chapter 5: Ideas for enhancing hospital social responsibility in Africa 177

    1. Recruiting and training the health workforce 177
    2. Providing leadership and governance 179
    3. Strengthening infrastructure and logistics 180
        1. Service delivery 181
        2. Health workforce (Caregivers) 183
        3. Information 184
    4. Providing medical products: The availability of medicines, cost control, equity of treatment: 185

    5. Securing financing: Funds and investments 188

    6. Providing leadership and governance (at the level of
       health authorities in African regions and countries) 189

Conclusion 191

Table of contents 215

www.ingramcontent.com/pod-product-compliance
Ingram Content Group UK Ltd.
Pitfield, Milton Keynes, MK11 3LW, UK
UKHW020858160426
5217IPUK00040B/1258